# Holistic Home

## CREATING AN ENVIRONMENT FOR SPIRITUAL AND PHYSICAL WELL-BEING

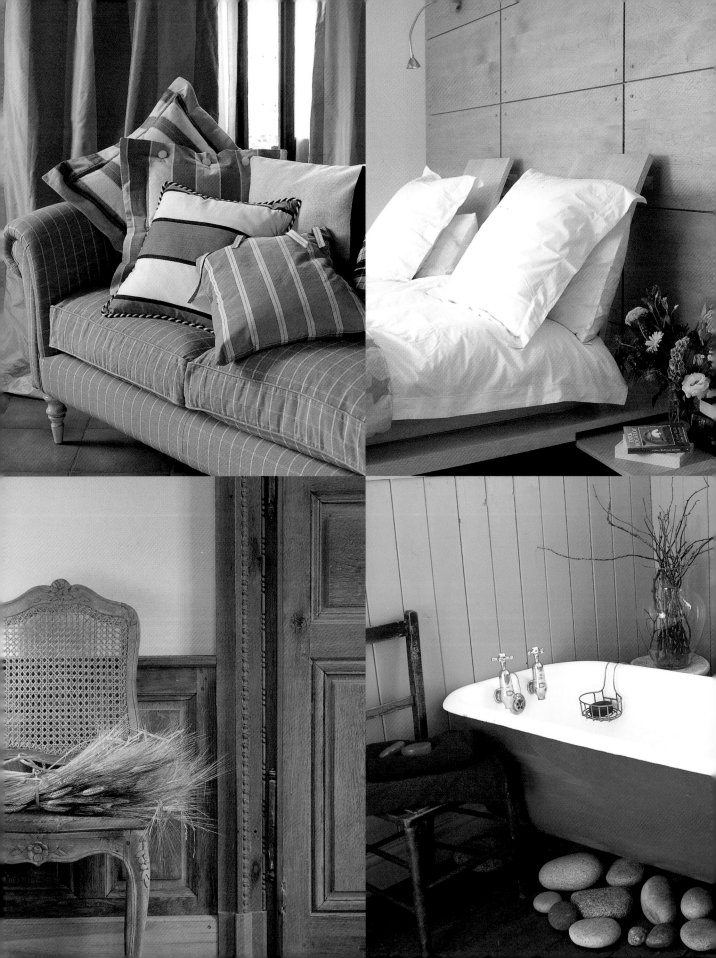

# Holistic Home

CREATING AN ENVIRONMENT FOR SPIRITUAL
AND PHYSICAL WELL-BEING

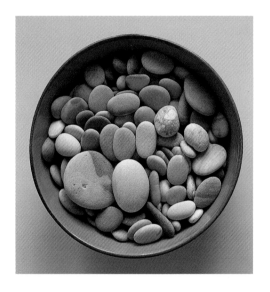

by Joanna Trevelyan

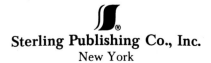

Sterling Publishing Co., Inc.
New York

A QUINTET BOOK

Library of Congress Cataloging-in-Publication Data is available on request

Published by Sterling Publishing Co., Inc.
387 Park Avenue South
New York, NY 10016-8810

Distributed in Canada by
Sterling Publishing
c/o Canadian Manda Group,
One Atlantic Avenue, Suite 105
Toronto, Ontario, Canada M6K 3E7

This book was designed and produced by
Quintet Publishing Limited
6 Blundell Street
London N7 9BH

CREATIVE DIRECTOR: Richard Dewing
DESIGNER: Isobel Gillan and Ian Hunt
PROJECT EDITOR: Lyn Coutts
MANAGING EDITOR: Diana Steedman
PHOTOGRAPHER: Paul Forrester

Typeset in Great Britain by
Central Southern Typesetters, Eastbourne
Manufactured in Singapore by United
Graphic Pte Ltd
Printed in Singapore by Star Standard
Industries Pte Ltd

ISBN 0-8069-1367-3

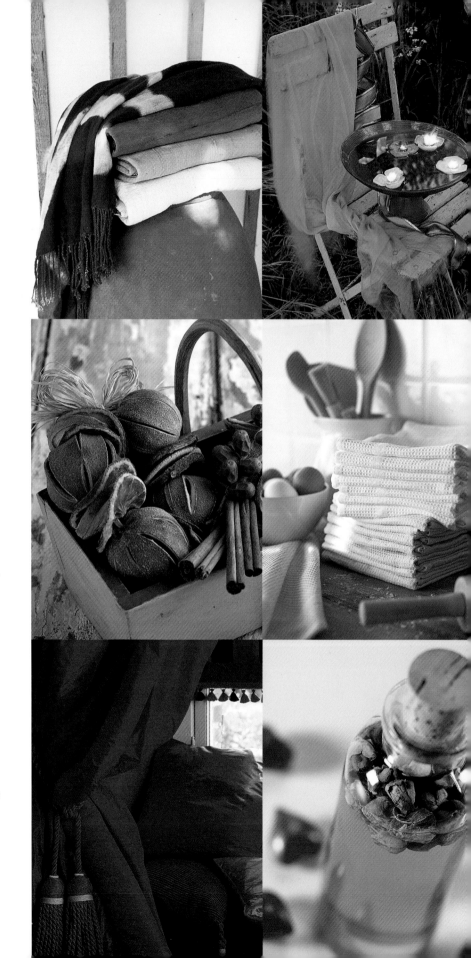

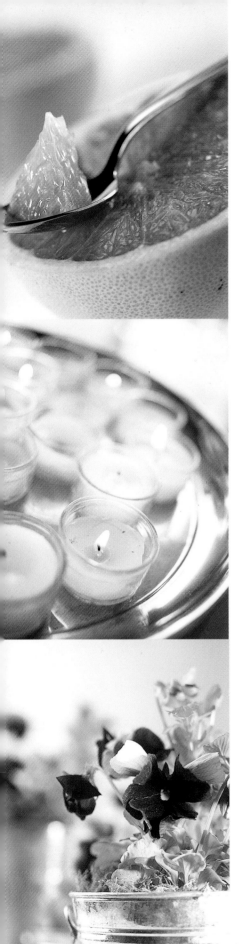

# Contents

# introduction

More and more people are looking for ways of improving the quality of their lives. The trend toward downshifting and more flexible working arrangements, the popularity of complementary therapies, and the widespread concern about pollution and the natural environment are examples of this new consciousness.

Few of us, however, are able to give up our nine-to-five job and urban existence for a natural wilderness and a self-supporting lifestyle. But the desire to make significant and life-long change has never been stronger.

This book provides the encouragement, inspiration, and information that will allow anyone—no matter where they live or what they do—to carry out simple and effective adaptations that will make their existing home truly holistic. And in making these changes to their physical environment, change will also be rendered to their health, and emotional and spiritual life.

What, though, does "holistic" mean? A dictionary definition is confusing rather than illuminating. A better model for a meaning comes from its practical application in health care. A holistic health practitioner takes into account the social, emotional, and spiritual concerns as well as physical and psychological ones of their patient. This all-encompassing definition, I believe, perfectly reflects what this book is about.

A home is more than just bricks and mortar—a physical barrier against the world. It should be seen as a second skin—a protective and nurturing envelope—that caters to your social needs for a welcoming meeting place for family and friends, and your psychological needs for rest, play, and study. A home has to be a sanctuary, a very personal place where your emotional and spiritual lives can be fulfilled, but at the same time it has to interact with the wider environment.

To fulfill such a wide brief, the holistic home is one that does more than provide warmth, shelter, and a place to hang your hat: it is a partner that has a positive impact on your health and well-being, and makes a contribution towards conserving the Earth's resources.

But that is not where change ends. By incorporating the principles of the ancient Chinese philosophy of feng shui into your home, you can manipulate ch'i (qi) energies to your advantage.

Each section of this book has a specific remit. The first section explores the principles and practicalities of holistic design and feng shui; the second is a room-by-room journey through your home and garden showing you how to use natural materials, color, texture, light, and scent. The final section is about an holistic lifestyle—looking after yourself, using complementary therapies, managing your time, and breaking the stress cycle.

The best thing about holism and feng shui is that the process of harmonizing your life with your immediate environment will not break the bank, nor will it send stress levels through the roof. On the contrary, you will only come to feel better and happier with every change you make. Why? Because you are making changes that will have positive effects for a lifetime.

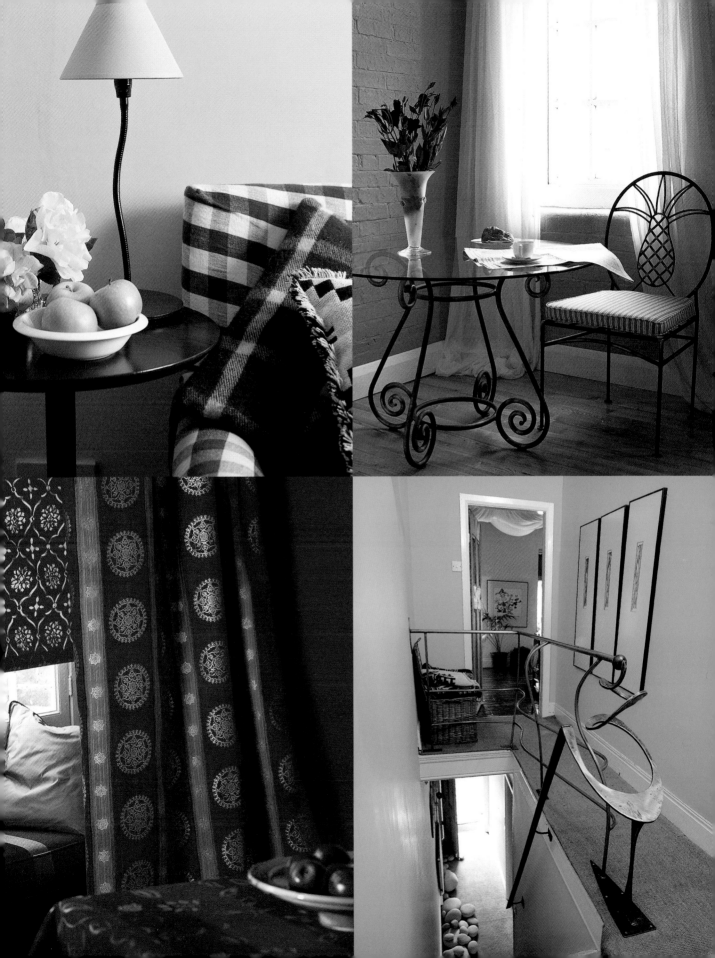

# CHAPTER 1
## *the* H O M E *sacred*

Since ancient times, people have recognized the sacredness of the home. As the center of life and a place of safety, it was vital that a home was built in an auspicious place and that the spirits believed to reside in it were appeased.

Many systems of house placement and design have developed with these aims in mind. There is, for example, the Hindu system of sacred siting called vastuvidya; the Chinese art of feng shui; and geomancy, a Western equivalent of feng shui.

Within the home, rites and rituals have been used for thousands of years to protect the household, to drive away evil or bad spirits, and to honor the spirit of the home. The Romans gave offerings of salt and flour to the home spirits, the Saxons fixed antlers to roof peaks to drive away evil, and Native American Indians planted a cactus at each corner of a home's foundations to guard against unwanted influences.

*Whether you use eucalyptus wreaths (LEFT) or corn sheaves (RIGHT), the clear message to evil spirits is "Keep out." A home in total harmony prevails (OPPOSITE).*

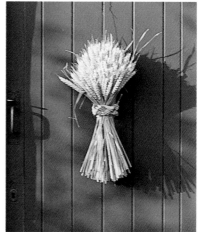

## *Cleansing*
### HARMONIZING

Many traditional cultures also believe in the importance of cleansing and harmonizing the energy of a home by undertaking purification rites when moving into a new home, at the change of the seasons, or after an illness or death has occurred. Whatever the ritual, the aim is to cleanse and heal the home, so that the occupants can live in peace and harmony. There is a very real sense in which the annual task of spring cleaning is a modern day, energy-cleansing ritual.

These rituals serve to remind us that the intimate relationship between ourselves, our homes, and our environment has been severed or made soul-less. Holistic design and feng shui can help you to reclaim this bond, filling your home with harmony and health so that it invigorates and not dulls the senses, and rekindles the embers of spirituality.

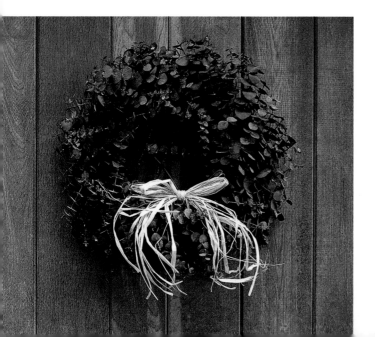

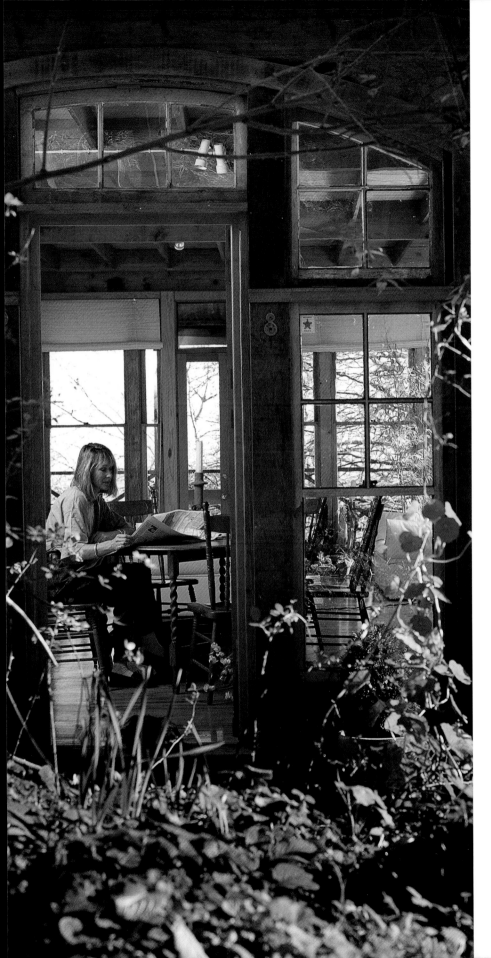

## CONTEMPORARY
*talismans*

*P*rotective talismans and rituals are still
in evidence today. Possibly the most
common is the horseshoe for luck. But
everything from leaves and thorns to
crossed knitting needles under the
doormat are in current use.

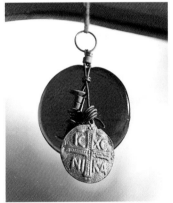

Pennsylvania Dutch hex symbols, first
brought to America by refugees from
Germany, are seen on the porches of
many American homes. These colorful,
round signs that incorporate symbols
like a dove, heart, star or rainbow
celebrate nature but also guard the
home. And it is a rare Greek home
that is not protected by the distinctive
blue eye (ABOVE). Some Greek
families carry on the tradition of
hanging a floral garland on the front
door on the first of May, and then
submitting the garland to the flames on
the same day in July. The garland is
burnt to destroy the bad spirits it has
absorbed while protecting the home. A
rope of garlic or onions hung in the
kitchen serves the same purpose, so woe
betide those who eat them!

## HOLISTIC DESIGN FOR HARMONIOUS LIVING

The key principle of holistic design is to do as little harm to ourselves and to the environment as possible. Hand-in-hand with this comes the inevitable improvement in the health of the home and its inhabitants. This is done by using natural, sustainable materials where possible; by excluding or reducing reliance on synthetic and potentially toxic products; and by looking at ways of conserving energy and other resources. Tackling these things, and at the same time bringing a little "magic" into the home with feng shui, harmonious colors, gentle lighting, welcoming sounds, heavenly smells, and flourishing plants will improve your home's subtle energies.

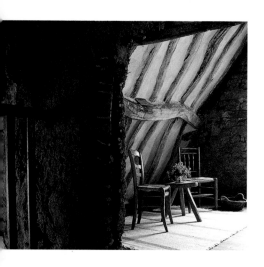

*A quiet hideaway in an old barn (LEFT), flooded with gentle light, bristling with fresh air, and devoid of modern artifice—a place of "magic."*

Every home has its own energies. Most of us have been in a place that we can't wait to leave. Conversely, we all know the wonderful feeling of being somewhere totally welcoming. These reactions are due to subtle energies—negative and unhealthy energies versus positive and healthy ones—flowing through a location.

Sick building syndrome is now recognized as a real problem, especially in modern high-rise offices that are virtually vacuum-sealed from the outside world. The combination of badly polluted air and drinking water, chemical emissions from synthetic building materials, and the effects of electrical equipment can lead to high levels of staff sickness. But just as debilitating are the blanket of even lighting, the shroud of a level-temperature environment, and open plan spaces devoid of character or personality. Our homes can also be sick, but there is a lot we can do to improve them.

A quick walk round your home is likely to reveal at least some of the following: wood treated with poisonous chemicals to prevent rot; old paint containing lead; synthetic carpets and furnishings; fumes and gases from open fires, unserviced cooking, cooling, and heating appliances; and cupboards full of chemical-based household cleaning products. Moreover, treated flooring, airtight windows, insulation foam, and layers of plastic (PVC) paint on the walls seal your home, trapping stale air and chemical vapors.

### Principles into practice

Before you throw yourself into redecorating, refurnishing or any major overhaul, ask what you want from your living space. It is helpful here to make a list of what your home means to you and what you need from it. Is it simply a place where you sleep and occasionally eat? Or is it a place where you work, entertain, and bring up your children? Does your home have to meet the needs of someone with a disability or an elderly person?

Alternatively, you can decide to start your holistic refurbishment in the most-used room in your home, or in a room that is vibrating with electrical equipment, choked with synthetic furnishings and fibers, and swooning under the fumes of petrochemical-based finishes.

Once your priorities are in place, detoxify the area as thoroughly as possible and strip or remove surfaces and items that are emitting noxious fumes. Give the area a spring clean and carry out a major sort to prune unnecessary clutter or energy-gobbling, noisy appliances. Then comes the really satisfying part—redesigning and redecorating to create an holistic living space.

It does not matter if the scale of your plans is modest or grand, an holistic home is one that evolves and improves with time. There will doubtless be compromises along the way—a heating or cooling system that cannot be renewed, replacement flooring that is beyond the budget, or pieces of furniture that just have to be tolerated. Do not let these setbacks stop you, since anything you do toward making your home an holistic one is beneficial.

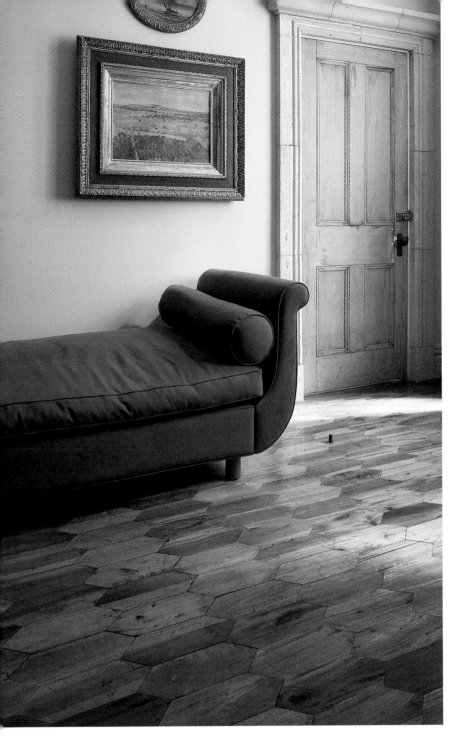

*Creating a harmonious whole with pleasing natural materials and careful placement of furniture is the essence of holistic and feng shui design.*

# Natural, sustainable
## MATERIALS

# A TOUCH OF
*magic*

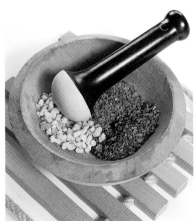

### Purification incense

*Mix together equal amounts of ground cedar, sandalwood, and myrrh in an earthenware or ceramic bowl. Burn the incense to counter any negativity.*

### Protection incense

*Combine the following ground ingredients in an earthenware or ceramic bowl: 1 part frankincense, 1 part myrrh, 1 part pine, ½ part basil, and ½ part sage. Burn the incense at the start or close of a day, at the beginning of a month or season, or after a significant event.*

### Cleansing mist

*Fill a spray mist container with spring water and add a few drops of Bach Rescue Remedy or Bach Wild Rose. The Rescue Remedy is particularly effective in clearing the after-effects of an argument and to cleanse a room where someone has been ill. To recreate a healthy, vital atmosphere, spray with Wild Rose mist.*

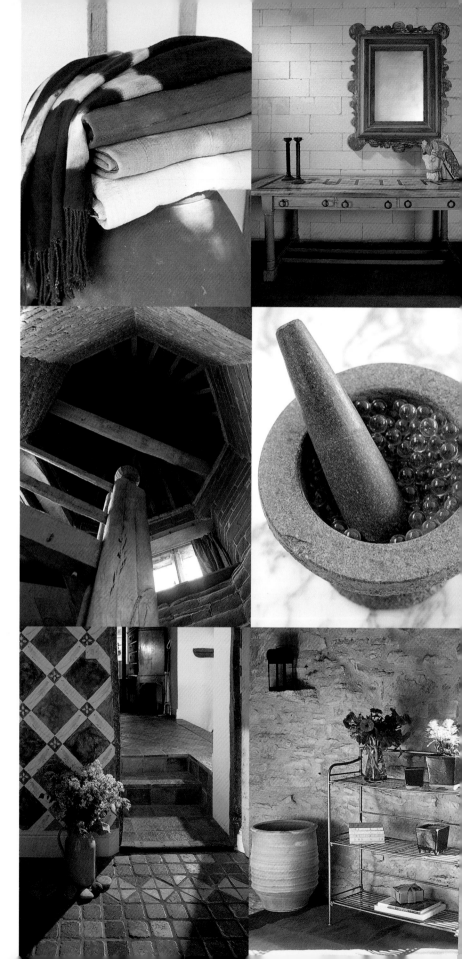

# BAUBIOLOGIE

*T*he Baubiologie—building biology— school of architecture has been developed in Europe, and aims to design and construct homes that fulfill all holistic requirements. Built with natural materials, these homes are compared with organisms. Their outer skin protects, insulates, absorbs, breathes, and communicates. Baubiologie homes are carefully sited to utilize sunlight and to avoid the negative effects of electromagnetic fields. Only energy- and resource-efficient systems are employed in the home.

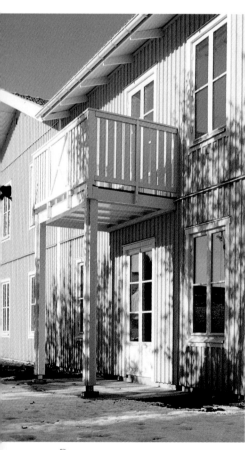

*B*alancing environmental, health and spiritual needs is the task of a natural home. If one element is sacrificed or dominated, the home will not be harmonious

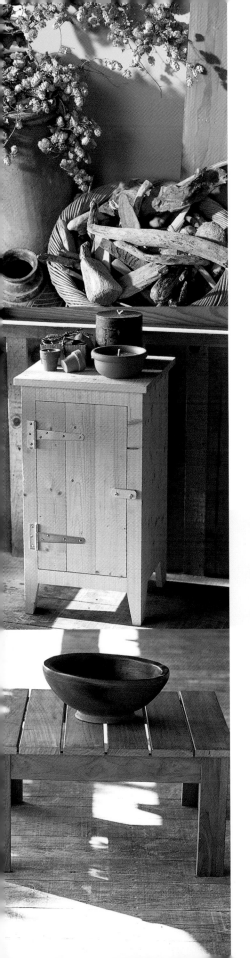

### Natural materials

Building and decorating with natural materials derived from sustainable or renewable sources, or even recycled, give pleasure beyond measure. They are a delight to the senses—their textures arouse and tickle your fingertips or toes, their colors warm and excite, and their scents evoke something that strikes your core. They also allow you to break the "tizzy-it-up" decorating mold, for when you are working with natural materials the inclination is to leave well enough alone. Why muddle with perfection?

Natural materials, though, come at a price. Some are derived from countries where economics is seen as more important than conservation, and others have been treated with toxic chemicals in order to fulfill importation criteria or perceived consumer requirements. The cost of surrounding yourself with natural materials is that you have to do some research. Be aware, for example, of timbers cut from threatened forests, or stone quarries that are disfiguring a landscape. Your background research will also help you to choose the right material for the right job.

*Materials from the natural world (LEFT) bring a beautiful simplicity to any home.*

> *"Before I built a wall I'd ask to know*
>
> *What I was walling in or walling out"*
>
> ROBERT FROST

There are two ideal places to find the natural decorating or building materials you need: the first is in a builder's reclamation yard, and the second is locally. Reclamation yards are springing up everywhere and even if you do not find what you need on your first reckoning, you are bound to on the second, third or fourth—trawling reclamation yards can become addictive. Locally manufactured or locally sourced materials means that gallons of gas have not been wasted transporting them around the country.

The fabric of your home uses lots of natural and healthy materials—glass, plaster, wood, stone, bricks, cement, and tiles. Lime plaster, for example, is a wonderful material. It is made using abundant natural resources, causes no health

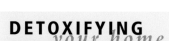

# DETOXIFYING
*your home*

| HAZARD | EFFECT | SOLUTION |
|---|---|---|
| Electromagnetic fields (EMFs) are generated by lights, household appliances, office equipment, and power lines running into the home. | Aggravate stress levels and trigger allergies. In extreme cases, increase the possibility of developing leukemia or a brain tumor. | Cut down use of electricity, remove electrical equipment from bedrooms, and sit further away from televisions and computers. EMF shields for computers can be purchased. Use an ionizer to generate negative ions, and improve ventilation and humidity. |
| Combustion gases such as gas, oil, paraffin, coal, and wood emit harmful by-products like carbon monoxide, formaldehyde, and sulfur dioxide. | Acute or prolonged exposure can cause, among other things, headaches and dizziness, and aggravate allergic reactions and respiratory problems. | Cookers, boilers, and heaters should be regularly serviced. Provide good ventilation, and have chimneys swept and checked for cracks. Replace a gas cooker with an environmentally cleaner and more efficient combustion stove. |
| Toxic vapors emitted by chemical-based cleaning products, paint, and decorating finishes. | Some of the chemicals can burn on contact with skin, cause nausea and worse if digested. A build-up of fumes will aggravate allergic reactions and respiratory problems. | Increase ventilation, and use natural ingredient-based cleaners (either proprietary brands or home-made), water-based paints tinted with natural pigments, and beeswax and linseed oil. |
| Formaldehyde vapors from synthetic household furnishings. | A potent irritant, which with prolonged inhalation can cause depression, headaches, and dizziness. | Replace with natural fabrics and upholstery fillings. |
| Old piping may be leaching lead, nitrates, and trace pollutants into the water supply. | Young children are extremely vulnerable, with absorption affecting the nervous system. Other effects: depression, fatigue, irritability, and stomach pains. | Replace lead piping or install an effective in-system water filter. Water filter jugs are inexpensive but the filter must be replaced regularly. |
| Air-borne bacteria and molds. | Symptoms among those with allergies include: coughing, breathing problems, nausea, and fever. | Air-conditioning units should be regularly checked, or install an air purification system. Increase cross-ventilation by opening windows and doors, or install a passive vent system. |
| Furniture, chairs, and bedding that do not correctly support the body. | Backache, poor sleep, and poor posture. Poorly designed office seating can cause tiredness. | Tackle the ergonomics of current furniture and bedding, and critically assess if chairs and sofas are firm enough to support your back and the base of the spine. Foot stools can help. A good bed should offer plenty of support for the spine while allowing hips and shoulders to lie comfortably. |
| Accumulated dirt and dust that may emit toxic or foul fumes, release mold and bacteria into the air, or prove hazardous for children or pets. | Increase likelihood of aggravating allergies or allergic reactions. In severe cases, inhalation or ingestion could result in poisoning. | Regular cleaning and a high standard of hygiene are critical. Pay particular attention to attics, roof areas, spaces behind kitchen units and electrical appliances, and basements. |

problems, and is non-polluting. Left in its natural state, unsmothered by petrochemical-based paint or vinyl (PVC) wallpaper, it breathes. It is the same with many other building and decorating materials—healthy and non-polluting in their raw state; but as toxic and unhealthy as synthetic products when treated or misused.

For example, wooden floorboards—old or new—need only a finish of linseed oil or beeswax to bring out the grain, to protect the wood, and to provide a safe surface for walking on. They do not need coats of synthetic stains or varnishes that contain volatile organic compounds and additives that emit unhealthy fumes. Certain dyes and dying processes, and stain-resist treatments, mean that natural fibers like cotton, linen, silk, and wool can give off toxic gases and cause allergic reactions. Instead, there are environmentally safe dying processes and naturally derived pigments.

The benefits of choosing natural materials over blended or synthetic ones are sometimes hard to assess, especially when buying carpets or rugs, for example. The only question you have to ask is: Would you wear it?

There is nothing short-term about using natural materials in your home. Nature's bounty never falls foul of any decorating trend—it survives them all—and natural materials get better with time and with use. Everyone has known the sensation of running their hand over an old newel post or stepping onto a worn and concave stone step. It is almost as though you are shaking the hand of everyone that has ever walked those stairs, or crossed that threshold.

### The three Rs—re-use, recycle, rethink

Not so long ago we threw away what we no longer needed. However, as more of us became aware of the enormity of the global waste disposal and pollution problem, seeking ways of reducing senseless waste and contributing to cleaning up our environment has became a priority.

Reducing waste by re-using (a home-centered operation that finds further uses for items) and recycling (the processing of manufactured products to provide the material to make new ones) are just two ways of making a personal contribution to a global problem.

Effective re-use and recycling means a reduced need for collection services, landfill sites, and for new products. These contribute to lessened pollution and land made unusable because of subsidence and toxic emissions.

Rethinking our patterns of consumption and manufacturing processes is the long-term goal that is only spurred on by the consumer. If consumer demand, for example, for a green product or process becomes great enough, then and only then will manufacturers invest the time and money to come up with an imaginative and environmentally sound alternative.

It is estimated that 80 percent of rubbish could be re-used in the same form, or recycled. Yet even in the most "green" countries only about 30 percent of glass containers are actually recycled. There is still a lot to do, but this is an area where individuals can make a difference.

*The knotted and stripped wood from an old door is given a second-lease of life in this kitchen unit (BELOW).*

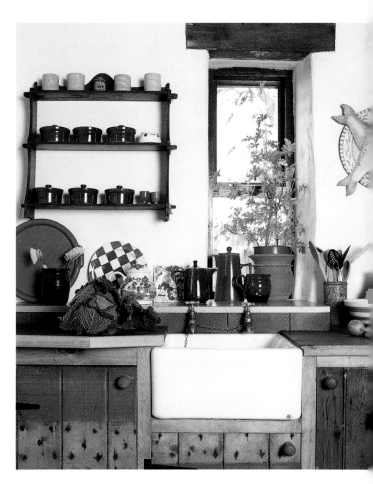

## THE ART OF FENG SHUI

Like holistic design, feng shui will help you to achieve a new look and a new way of living.

Feng shui—meaning "wind and water"—is derived from the ancient Chinese principle of siting temples and homes in locations where the elements were in harmony, and where they would be protected from wind but near a source of fresh water. It was much later that feng shui was used to manipulate surroundings in order to divine a home that promotes health, wealth, and happiness.

Feng shui taps into many aspects of Chinese culture: the tao, yin/yang theory, Chinese astrology, I ching, and so on. Since "feng" refers to moving air, it readily conjures up the idea of ch'i or qi—the energy that animates all of nature. The essence of feng shui is to harmonize the three types of ch'i energy. These energies are found in the atmosphere, in the land, and in the human body. It is the ch'i in the body that acupuncturists seek to regulate and enhance.

### The different energies

Ch'i or qi—the subtle flow of energy through everything in the universe. Feng shui manipulates ch'i so that it flows harmoniously from one thing or one place to another. A distinctive type of ch'i energy is found in different "sectors" of the home. These sectors are distinguished by their direction (which is determined with a compass) from the physical center of the home.

Yin/yang—these are two kinds of ch'i energy—yin being passive, and yang, active. Their meanings were extended to express the delicate balance of dark (yin) and light (yang).

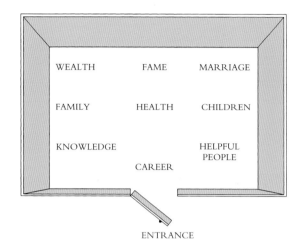

| WEALTH | FAME | MARRIAGE |
| FAMILY | HEALTH | CHILDREN |
| KNOWLEDGE | | HELPFUL PEOPLE |
| | CAREER | |

ENTRANCE

*Orientate the ba-gua chart so that the entrance to the room (see label) aligns with the main door into a room. To apply this to a desk or similar, align the entrance with your seating position.*

Nothing is ever purely yin or purely yang: there is always an element of each in both. This is clearly depicted in the yin/yang symbol.

Because elements in the home are attributed with different yin and yang qualities, they can be used to alter ch'i. For example, the shady side of your home is more yin, while the sunny side is more yang. On the basis of this, you can determine the most appropriate activities for particular rooms that will balance the two energies.

I ching—this is the ancient Chinese book of divination and philosophy from which the nine trigrams (ba-gua) are sourced. In feng shui, the ba-gua grid is laid over maps, floor plans of a home or room, or scale drawings of a desk or workstation, in order to relate specific areas with the unique qualities of the nine trigrams. These qualities are fame, marriage, children, helpful people, career, knowledge, family, wealth, and health. It is by diagnosing and adjusting the ch'i in these areas that feng shui can offer help with specific problems.

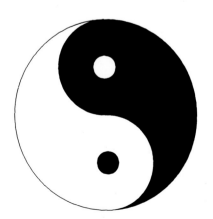

*The yin/yang symbol expresses the delicate balance of nature.*

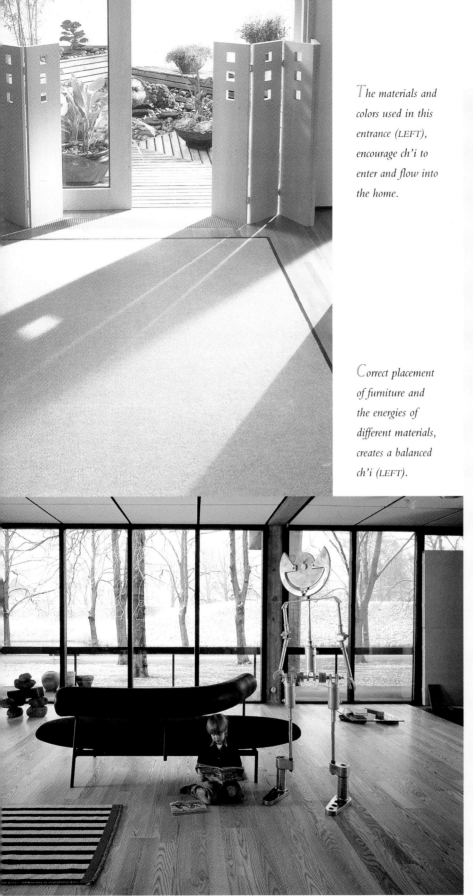

*The materials and colors used in this entrance (LEFT), encourage ch'i to enter and flow into the home.*

*Correct placement of furniture and the energies of different materials, creates a balanced ch'i (LEFT).*

# FIVE *elements*

*E*ach element describes a certain type of ch'i energy that is linked to a season and direction, and to materials, shapes, and colors.

Tree element is associated with growth and vitality—spring; east/south-east; timber; vertical and rectangular; green.

Fire element is associated with passion and warmth—summer; south; plastic (though this material has a negative effect on ch'i) and metal; pointed and triangular; red.

Earth element is associated with comfort and security—late summer; natural fibers, plaster, ceramics, bricks; horizontal and squat; yellow and brown.

Metal element is associated with richness and leadership—fall; west; metals and hard stone; round; white, gold, and silver.

Water element is associated with tranquility and power—winter; north; glass; organic, irregular shapes; black.

These energies will help you use a room or home's aspects most favorably, or will indicate how to manipulate furniture and decoration to correct unfavorable energies. For example, a room's fire ch'i energy can be increased with star-print fabric or decoration; white will enhance metal ch'i energy; and natural fibers will strengthen earth (sometimes called soil) energy.

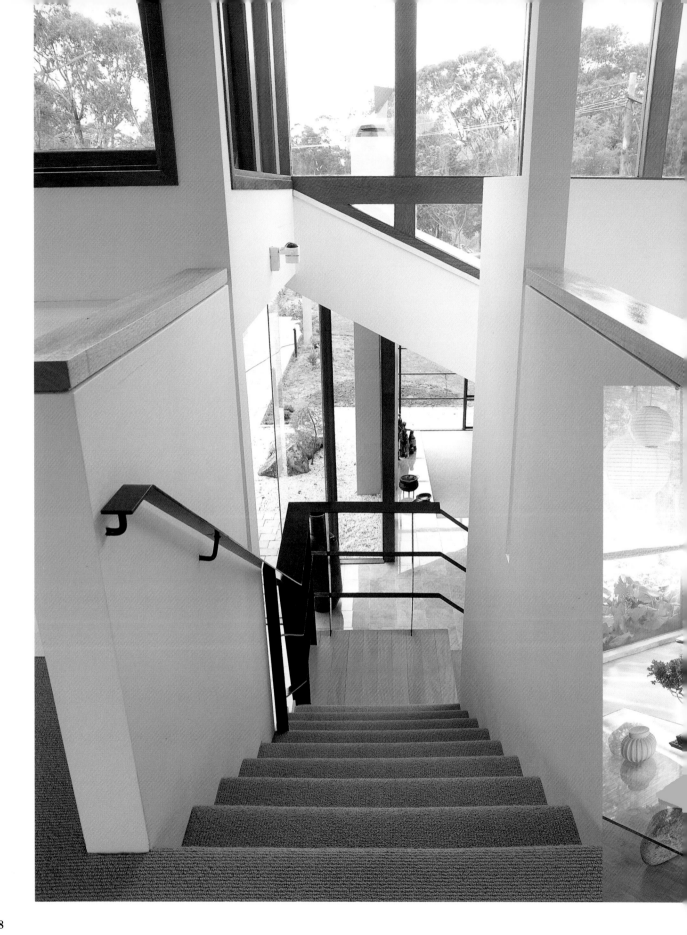

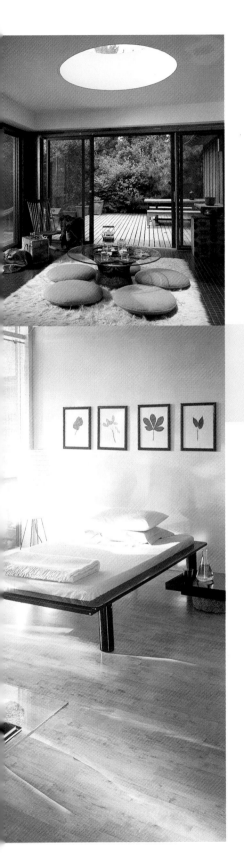

### Philosophy into practice

You can use feng shui to find the ideal site for a home, or to remedy unfavorable ch'i. In feng shui terms, the ideal is a home sited on the south side of a hill, with the hill rising up behind the home. A gentle slope should run from the front of the home down to a stream. But if your home—like most—is not so idyllically positioned, the ch'i can be corrected by using trees, pathways and driveways, lighting, and garden features like a pond or waterfall.

To assess the flow of ch'i within a building, draw an accurate floor plan of the home, doing one for each floor of a multi-storey construction, that includes all internal walls, doors, windows, staircases, fireplaces, and fixed items (stove, oven, baths, and toilets, for example). Also indicate features

*Stampeding ch'i in a light-filled, entrance (FAR LEFT), is slowed by ceramic pots and sculptures and sisal runners.*

*"It was chance which made men turn gold into their symbol, rather than stone"*

### VITA SACKVILLE-WEST

like overhead beams, supporting pillars or sloping roofs that will hinder the flow of ch'i.

Use a ruler to find the physical center of the home, and of all the main rooms. A compass will let you determine the direction the home and the relative position of each room within.

These floor plans let you work out the most favorable use and layout of a room according to the ch'i energies of the five elements or the ba-gua.

To work out the ba-gua, simply trace the ba-gua grid onto semi-transparent paper and lay it over the floor plan. The door opening on the grid must align with the main door into the home or into the room.

*Every item from paper lamps to tables mounted on stones (LEFT) helps to balance ch'i in this restful bedroom. (ABOVE LEFT) Eastern influences, maintain the energies in this convivial setting.*

## *Passion*
### EXPRESSIVENESS

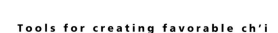

**Tools for creating favorable ch'i**

Ch'i energy should enter the home through the main entrance, flow smoothly throughout each area, and then exit somewhere near to its point of entry. Everything in the home will affect how and where the ch'i moves. Walls may block it, mirrors deflect it, recesses stagnate it, sisal or rush flooring slow it, and glass may cause it to stampede or move too quickly.

These problems can be corrected to create favorable ch'i movement by using the following tools.

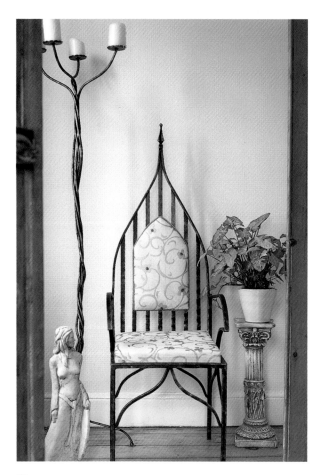

*T*all, *black wrought iron candle holders are associated with the soil and metal energies.*

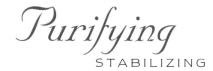

*Purifying*
STABILIZING

◆ *Candles*—these bring fire ch'i energy to an area, and encourage passion and expressiveness. They are also helpful in rooms that lack natural sunlight and may be filled with stagnant ch'i. The effect of a candle depends on its color.

◆ *Crystals*—these will enhance and disperse ch'i in specific areas. A student, for example, can exaggerate the energy in the knowledge sector of a room by hanging a quartz crystal in that area.

◆ *Decorating and building materials*—each material brings with it a different sort of ch'i energy. Wood is neutral in its effect, whereas glass and metal encourage ch'i energy to move faster. Plant fibers such as sisal and rush slow ch'i, as do ceramics and clay. The color of the material will also influence ch'i. Plastics block ch'i and their use should be avoided .

◆ *Mirrors*—these have many uses, which is why they are referred to as "the aspirin" of feng shui. Use mirrors to reflect threatening ch'i and to stimulate good ch'i.

◆ *Plants*—use to move nourishing ch'i throughout a room, and to blunt acute angles that jut into a room and cut ch'i energy.

◆ *Sculptures and rocks*—use heavy objects to stabilize an unsettled situation in any of the ba-gua positions. A sculpture in the career sector of a room might help a person worried about their job prospects, for example.

◆ *Sea salt*—this is the most yang of foods, and it attracts ch'i energy that has a purifying and stabilizing influence.

◆ *Water fountain or aquarium*—these are a symbol of money and will therefore stimulate ch'i in the wealth or career sector of a home. Moving water also enhances ch'i.

◆ *Wind chimes*—will bring positive ch'i into a room that is deficient in ch'i, or will moderate the flow of ch'i if hung near an entrance. Ch'i is stimulated by vibrating air, so in place of wind chimes you can also use chiming clocks or bells.

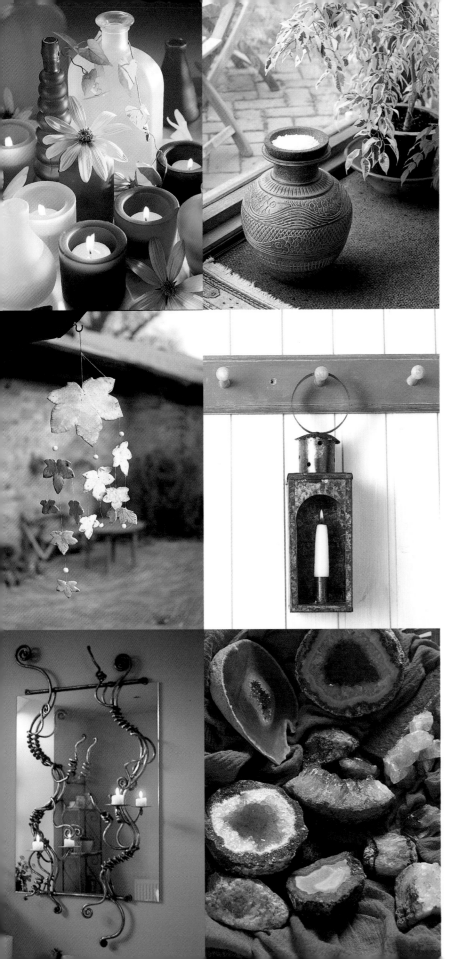

## CRYSTALS *crystalized*

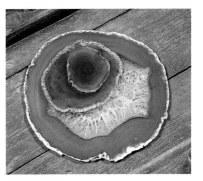

*Q*uartz crystals are used in healing rituals, and are thought to be able to maintain the energy and vitality of a home. In feng shui, crystals are hung in a window to attract ch'i energy into dark or stagnant areas of a room. Many people select their crystals by running their finger over a selection, and choosing the ones that seemingly pull at their finger or "talk to them." You can dedicate a crystal to maintaining the health, peace, and happiness of your home.

Crystals must be cleansed regularly, either by placing them on a piece of silk in the Sun, or by soaking the crystal for one or two days in a cup of water to which ½ cup of sea salt or table salt has been added.

*F*eng shui solutions for bad ch'i: candles, sea salt, wind chime, mirror, crystals, in settings that include glass, ceramic, stone, clay, wood, and metal.

# 2 *color*

C olor has a profound impact on our lives, and even the blind are known to experience colors through their fingers. In describing an object, we first define it by its color; when buying clothes or furnishings, it is usually a particular color that we seek; and it is color that we use when trying to express our personality and mood. This preoccupation with color is not a new thing, it is as old as civilization itself. Color "speaks", therefore it is not surprising that every culture has devised ways of using what can only be described as a very powerful language.

The ancient Egyptians diagnosed some illnesses as being due in part to color imbalances. They treated the patient by bathing them in the deficient color. Healing amulets and talismans were also painted in specific colors to suit the purposes for which the charms were being evoked.

The role of color in healing persists and thrives today. There are those who claim to be able to see an aura of glowing colors surrounding all living things. A healthy person is said to have a bluish aura with a balanced spectrum of colors, while an ill person has an aura in which color and shape changes.

In medieval Europe, nine colors were used in heraldic crests, and each color had a symbolic meaning. Yellow or gold for honor and loyalty; white or silver, faith and purity; red, courage; blue, piety and resolution; black, mourning and grief; green, youth and vitality; purple, high rank; orange, strength and endurance; and violet or amethyst, passion and suffering.

Earlier we briefly mentioned Pennsylvanian Dutch hex symbols, but it is not just the symbols that are imbued with meaning—their color is equally significant. Green is believed to bring happiness, luck and prosperity to the home; blue

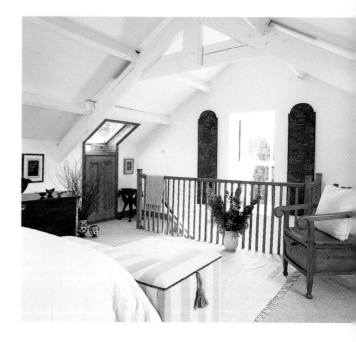

*N*eutral colors (ABOVE) are a background to the palette of wood tones that dominate this invitingly calm bedroom.

symbolizes spiritual love, protection, beauty and truth; brown is the earth color and evokes sensual pleasure; red heralds love and liberty; and white, purity, joy and protection. A combination of blue, red, and yellow is a guard against sickness and spells.

We still associate these colors with similar sentiments, and when we look at other cultures, both ancient and modern, there are many parallels—white for purity, red for danger, black for death. There are exceptions, however—for instance, in China white is a mourning color: the overriding message is that the effect of color is profound.

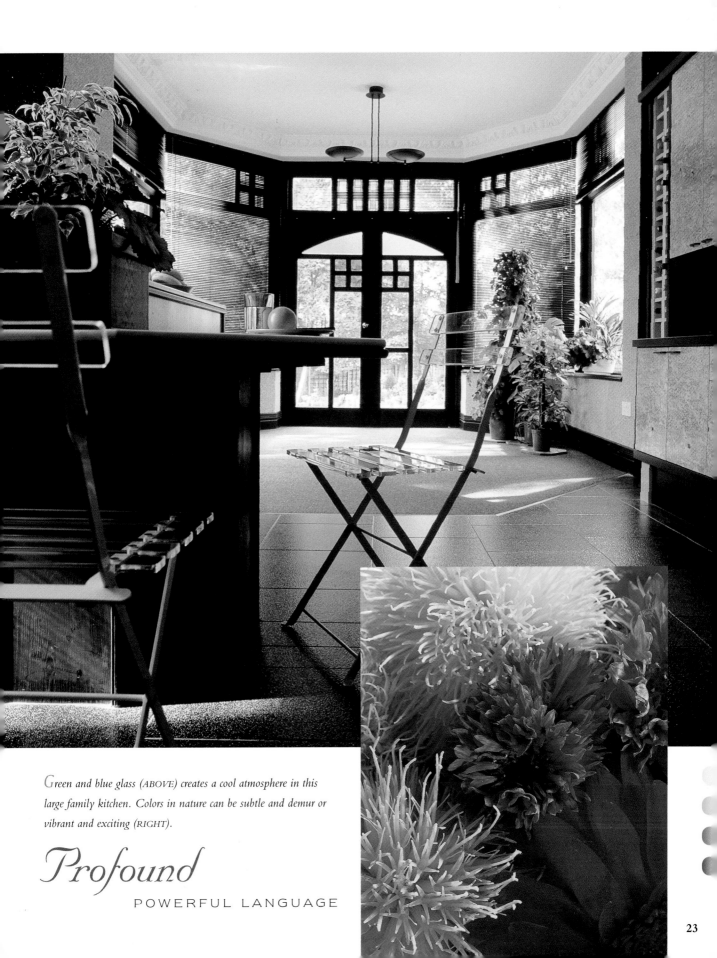

*G*reen and blue glass (ABOVE) creates a cool atmosphere in this large family kitchen. Colors in nature can be subtle and demur or vibrant and exciting (RIGHT).

# *Profound*
## POWERFUL LANGUAGE

## HOW COLORS AFFECT US

At a very basic level, most of us have color preferences—our favorites and the ones we detest. But color also affects us at a much deeper level. We can see this influence in the way we use color to describe how we feel—"I saw red", "I'm green with envy", or "I'm feeling blue". These simple, everyday turns of phrase underline truths borne out by scientific and psychological research.

We now know that exposure to the warm colors (red, orange, and yellow) increases our blood pressure, pulse, and respiratory rate, while exposure to cool colors (green, blue, and black) has the opposite effect. So when architects changed the color of school room walls in America from orange and white to blue, students' blood pressure dropped, and good behavior and learning comprehension soared.

Children with attention deficit disorder seem to be calmer in brightly colored rooms, whereas children with learning disabilities do best in rooms decorated in cool colors such as blue, green or gray. Color affects not only children, but also adults as the following example shows. In American correction centers, inmates are put in pink rooms to calm

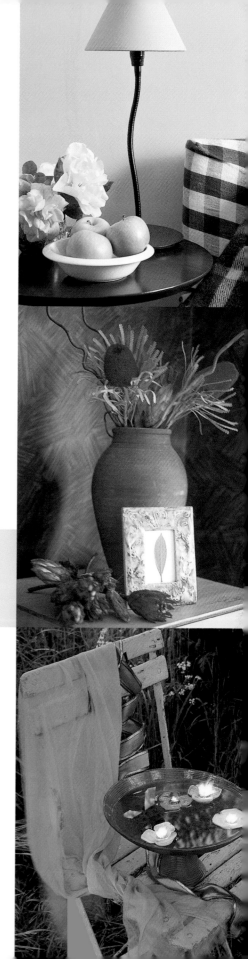

*All the colors of the rainbow (RIGHT): use them well and your home will bring you as much pleasure as those magical arches in the sky.*

> *"The purest and most thoughtful minds are those which love colour the most"*
>
> JOHN RUSKIN

them, rather than sedated with drugs. Pink apparently calms even the most aggressive prisoner within minutes.

Color is capable of setting up what have been described as "responsive vibrations." Thus people who are blind have been found to be able to perceive certain colors through touch. Red has been described as warm, rough, and tingling; and blue as smooth and cool, by severely visually impaired participants in Russian research studies—even when the temperature and texture of the surfaces touched were exactly the same. It seems clear from such studies that color not only affects us visually, but also at other energetic levels. With so much at stake, no wonder the task of choosing decorating colors can take so long!

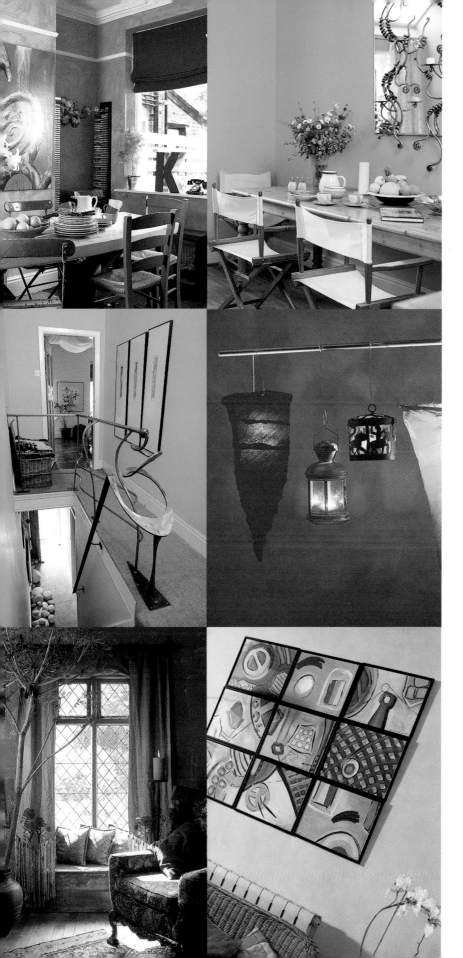

# COLOR *therapy*

*C*olor therapists use a simple color preference assessment to explore an individual's personality and state of mind. The therapist offers color advice to the client that will foster self-awareness and allow the client to maintain a balanced and harmonious life. Color therapy is also used in association with color counseling, to help relieve emotional disturbances and psychological imbalances.

✦ COLOR IS USED TO TREAT SPECIFIC DISEASES. YELLOW, FOR EXAMPLE, IS SAID TO ACTIVATE THE MOTOR NERVES AND GENERATE ENERGY FOR MUSCLES; THEREFORE A COLOR THERAPIST WILL EMPLOY IT TO TREAT ARTHRITIS, RHEUMATISM, DIGESTIVE PROBLEMS, ECZEMA, AND CONSTIPATION, FOR EXAMPLE.

✦ SURGEONS AND OTHER HEALTH PROFESSIONALS OFTEN WEAR GREEN GOWNS. COULD THIS BE BECAUSE GREEN IS BELIEVED TO INSPIRE HOPE AND PROMOTE HEALING?

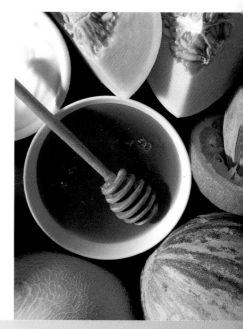

## NATURE'S PALETTE

The subtlety of hue and shade in natural materials is astounding, almost daunting if you take the time to look closely. In a handful of shells or pebbles you can find washed-out and strident shades of white, cream, yellow, gray, fawn, pink, tan, charcoal, and black.

Looking at color in nature is the best way of determining what you might like in your home. What you like looking at—whether it is fields of grain, the sea, a coppice of trees, gathering clouds, whatever—gives a hint as to the sort of colors, and even textures, that you might like to surround yourself with. And as the Sun moves high and low, and dips behind a cloud, you can also see how colors are mutated by light.

Choosing a color is very personal, and finding the exact hue or shade is a journey you must take alone.

*You can find color inspiration in the most surprising places—while preparing a meal (RIGHT) or creatively arranging a vase of Icelandic poppies (BELOW).*

### Warm colors

*Where to use*—kitchen, dining room, living room.

*How to use*—warm colors advance, tending to make them dominate cool colors and neutrals.

## FENG SHUI AND COLOR

Every color affects ch'i energy differently, and because of this colors are believed to be related to yin/yang and the five elements. Color can be used to maintain, calm and enhance a specific ch'i energy. Red, for example, is the most yang color and is linked with fire energy and the ch'i energy of the west.

Colors also have symbolic meanings. Red is associated with romance, wealth, and happiness. Three good reasons why the Chinese choose red for doors and entrance arches.

In essence, feng shui uses colors in two ways—two ways that are not totally dissimilar to our current use of color in the home. Large areas, or backgrounds, tend to be pale. Accent colors, which are more vivid, are used more sparingly on only small surfaces, such as a piece of furniture. The principle is: the stronger the color, the less is needed for it to be effective.

Personal preference is considered important in feng shui, so it is unwise to use a color, even if highly favorable and auspicious, if you do not actually like it.

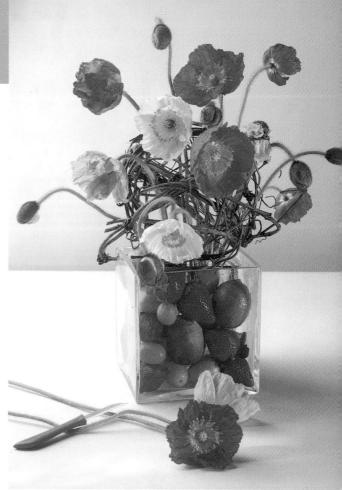

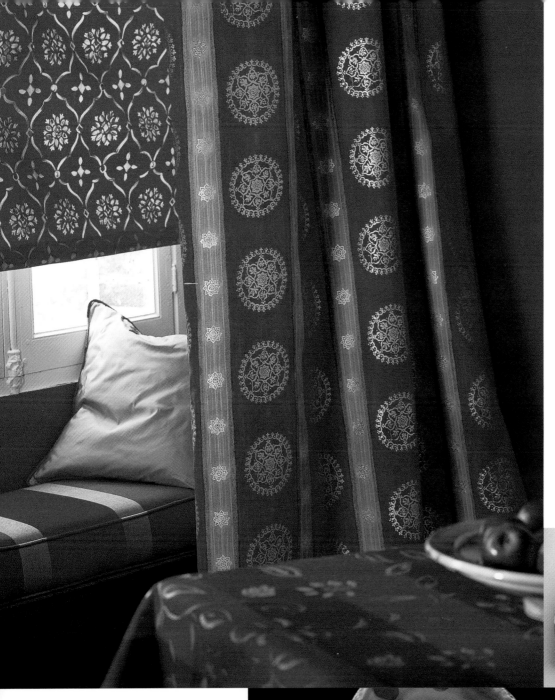

*Glowing yellows and oranges invite you to feel social and optimistic (LEFT), while the red excites passion.*

*Use the colors of a simple shell (BELOW) to create a color scheme for a whole room.*

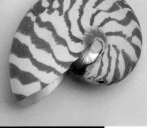

*Rings of amber yellow and fiery orange merge and dissolve into each other in this crystal (RIGHT).*

*Insight*
CREATIVITY

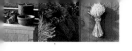

*A neutral background with electrifying red accents (RIGHT) perfectly illustrates a feng shui use of color.*

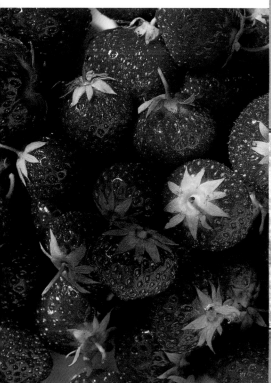

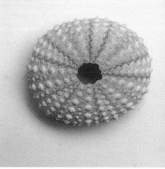

*Take your cue from nature (TOP AND ABOVE) when it comes to shades of reds and pinks.*

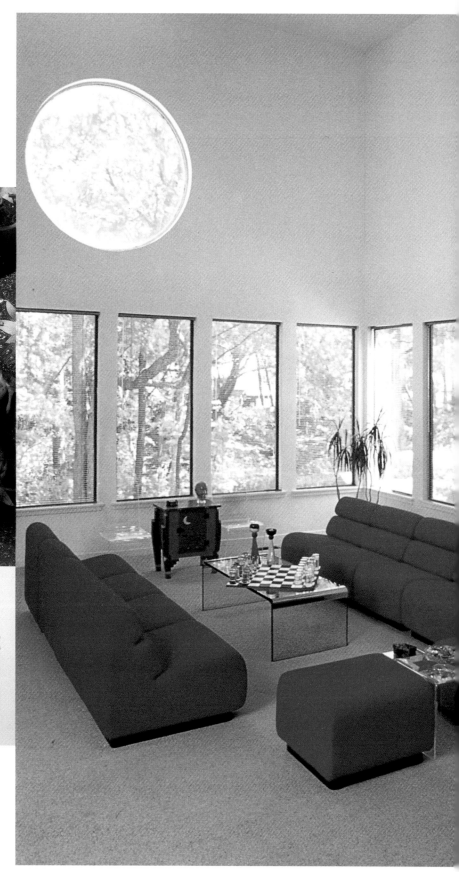

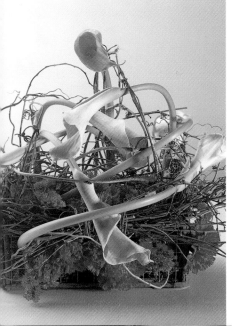

*A* floral decoration that will add a sense of joy and contentment to a room (LEFT).

*A* windowsill arrangement (BELOW) that is as emotionally healing as the scene beyond.

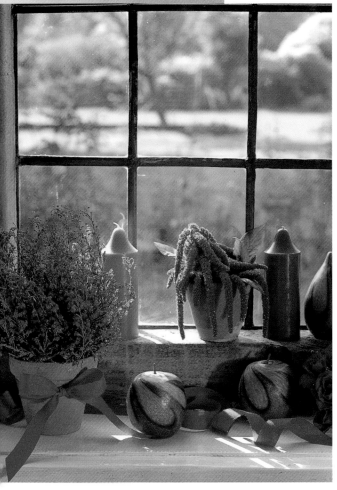

## Uplifting yellows

Associated with good luck and can stimulate joy, wisdom, intuitive insight, and creativity. It is a color that encourages flexibility and adaptability. Yellow can lift your mood, inspire optimism, and improve your sense of well-being. Color therapists claim it also has a positive effect on the nervous system and gastrointestinal tract. In excess, yellow can overstimulate and irritate, and is also associated with negative sentiments such as cowardice and prejudice. Creamy or pale-earth yellows create an illusion of space in a vista where pokiness once reigned, and citrus yellows will accentuate natural available light.

## Extrovert orange

A happy, social color that animates feelings of optimism, confidence, and enthusiasm. It will prickle creativity, ambition, and energetic activity. It is used by color therapists to treat a range of problems including asthma, colds, thyroid problems, and even to stimulate lactation. In some people, however, orange can produce nervousness and restless behavior.

## Passionate reds

Stimulate the senses and are associated with strength, joy, motivation, and love. This energy translates into an exciting and courageous decorating color. In color therapy it is used as a tonic, to improve blood circulation, and to overcome depression, fear, and inertia.

Attention-seeking reds must also be used carefully. They can generate fear, uncontrolled passion, and excessive anger, and may be disturbing to those with mental health problems or neuroses.

## Plucky pinks

Magenta hues signify spiritual completeness and sense of contentment. In all strengths, pink is a symbol of self-respect and self-awareness, but some people may find it mentally draining. It is regarded as the color of "universal healing" because it can raise the vibrations or energies of the body.

## "GREEN" ALTERNATIVES

The manufacture of many color pigments involves the use of non-renewable petrochemical and mineral resources. Moreover, paint-manufacturing processes can lead to pollution of the atmosphere and the water supply. To adequately dilute the paint that washes off a paintbrush so that it causes no environmental hazard, would require leaving the tap running for several days!

Conventional synthetic paints and other finishes, also give off noxious fumes even when dry. The concoction of chemicals, preservatives, fungicides, and pesticides can cause allergic reactions or respiratory problems. The long-term health problems associated with paint containing lead, for example, are only now being fully appreciated. To avoid damaging your health and causing further damage to the environment, it is worth considering using water-dilutable

*Earth colors are warming and work well in living rooms (RIGHT).*

*Put away the color charts and scour your store cupboard and garden for earthy color combinations (BELOW AND BOTTOM RIGHT).*

> *"The clouds that gather round the setting sun*
> *Do take a sober colouring ..."*
>
> WILLIAM WORDSWORTH

paints made from plant oils, resins, and waxes that are colored with sustainable earth, mineral, and plant pigments. These products give a wonderful finish but it is important that you read-up on how best to use and apply them.

There are also environmentally healthy alternatives to wood varnishes and stains, mineral spirits, and even floor and furniture waxes. It is surprisingly easy to make paint or to concoct a beeswax, herb, and linseed oil polish in your very own kitchen.

Before you start mixing up a paint or slapping on a conventional surface treatment, it is worth remembering that materials such as wood, clay, stone, and lime plaster are naturally imbued with color, and do not necessarily require painting. The tendency to coat all surfaces puts a barrier between a material's texture, resonance, and smell and you. Left in their raw state or given a minimal protective finish, natural materials can provide a color scheme—harmonious in every respect—that can be the basis of your redecorating.

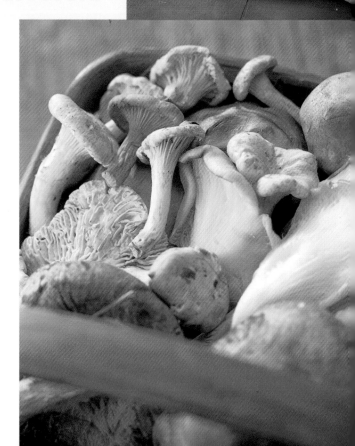

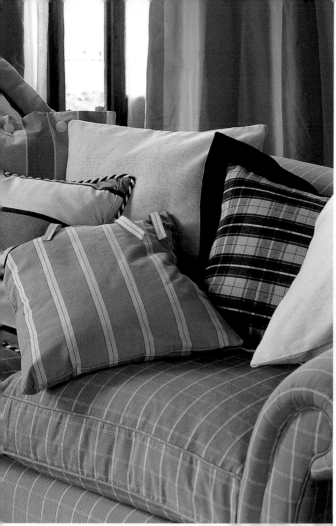

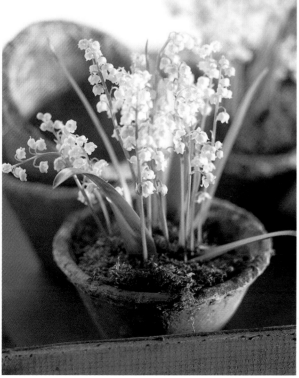

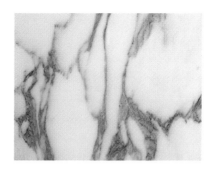

*Whites are found in nature tinted with other colors (LEFT). Follow nature's lead to avoid expanses of sterile white.*

### Neutrals and earth colors

*Where to use*—neutrals and pale earth tones have a unifying influence that works well in halls and entrances, but because they are easy on the eye and easy to live with, they can be used almost anywhere.

*How to use*—Strong earth colors should be treated as warm colors.

### Pure white

White blends all the rainbow colors, and represents harmony and purity. White is a revealer of truth and can lead us toward higher spiritual and divine knowledge. The Druids, an ancient tribe of Britain, regarded white as a symbol of the Sun and light, their priests wearing white in deference to this. In excess, however, white can feel unfriendly, sterile, and unapproachable. White with tints of warm or cool colors better represents the tones of white found in nature.

### Earth colors

Represent fertility, are associated with the environment and things in their natural state, and are said to dispel mental depression. Brown is a homeostatic, or balancing, color that creates a sense of security, although in excess it can extinguish a sense of vitality.

### Basic black

Associated with death and grief, but also with mystery and the unknown. It is an inward-looking color, absorbing and silent. Used with care it can be dramatic and powerful, and heighten emotions, but in excess it may be overwhelming or depressing, soaking up energy and vitality.

31

## TANTALIZING
### *all the senses*

*A*n holistic home will invigorate all the senses—sight, hearing, smell, touch, and even taste once you've swopped hermetically-sealed, ready-made foods for tasty, seasonal, organic produce, and lots of home cooking. It is therefore an environment that is especially suited to the sensory needs of babies and young children, older people, the infirm, and people with disabilities. For not only is it a healthy environment but holism addresses psychological, emotional, and spiritual desires to see, touch or smell lovely things, or to hear only the sweetest sounds.

The following ideas will help you to make your home a special delight for people with disabilities.

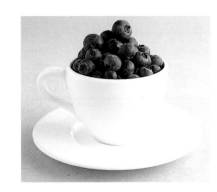

*A* combination of greens and blues (BELOW) creates a sense of harmony and calm that makes relaxation inevitable.

✦ FOR THE VISUALLY IMPAIRED—AROMA, TEXTURE, AND SOUND ARE CRITICAL, BUT COLOR SHOULD NOT BE DISREGARDED AS EVIDENCE SHOWS THAT COLOR CAN BE PERCEIVED THROUGH TOUCH. FILL THE AIR WITH POTPOURRIS AND SCENTED PLANTS TO LIFT THE MOOD; AND TO ACT AS SIGNPOSTS FOR CERTAIN ROOMS, PIECES OF FURNITURE, AND THE LOCATION OF A TELEPHONE AND THE LIKE. WIND CHIMES, BELLS, AND BURBLING INDOOR WATER FEATURES MAKE WELCOME COMPANY. FABRICS AND FURNITURE, FLOORING AND RUGS, PLANTS AND OBJECTS WITH INTERESTING AND VARIED TEXTURES WILL STIMULATE AND EDUCATE VIA THE FINGERTIPS.

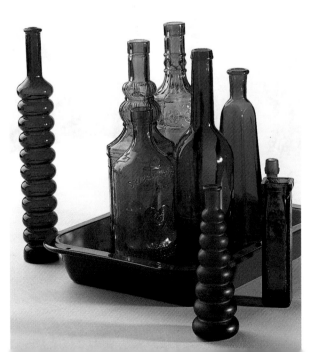

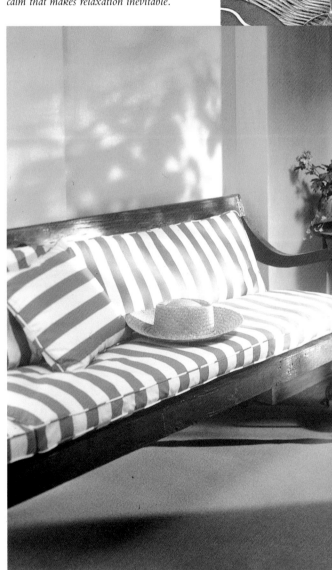

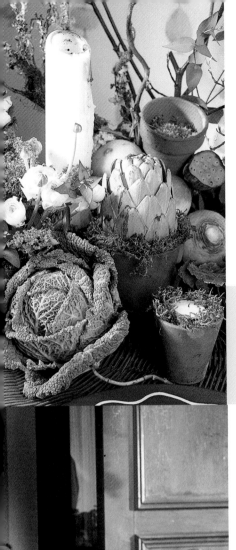

### Crisp greens

Sitting on the cusp between the warm and cool colors, green offers a sense of balance, that can exhibit itself in indecision. Green reminds us of the abundance of nature and is both restful and energizing. Green is closely linked to healing, and color therapists use it to soothe pain. On the negative side, it is a symbol of selfishness, jealousy, and laziness. Too much green can be depressing and debilitating.

*Images that encapsulate the meaning of two colors: soothing blue (FAR LEFT) and energizing green (LEFT).*

### Cool colors

**Where to use**—bedrooms, bathrooms, meditation and therapy rooms.

**How to use**—cool colors recede and can give an illusion of space.

### Mellow blues

Soothing and sedating, blues generate a sense of hope, harmony and calm. Blue can also stimulate creativity, communication, and spiritual understanding. Color therapists use it as a tonic, and say it has antiseptic qualities. Research also suggests it may be effective in guided imagery therapies to reduce pain levels. Blue has been used successfully in mental institutions to calm violent patients. In excess, blue may be depressing.

*Use details to introduce green (BELOW) and blue (FAR LEFT) into the home.*

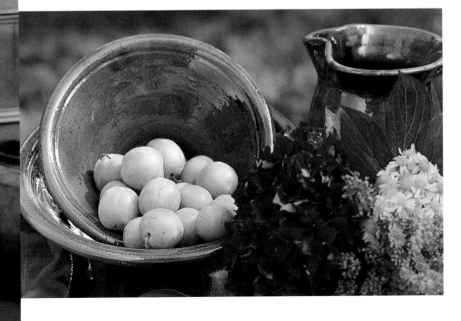

◆ FOR THE HEARING-IMPAIRED—COLOR, SMELL, AND TEXTURE SHOULD BE STRESSED BUT OBJECTS LIKE SHINY, METAL WIND CHIMES THAT MOVE AND GLINT IN RESPONSE TO WIND SHOULD ALSO BE USED.

◆ FOR THE PHYSICALLY-DISABLED—ALTHOUGH PRACTICAL CONSIDERATIONS OFTEN DICTATE WHERE FURNITURE IS PLACED, THE EMPHASIS ON CLEAR AND UNCLUTTERED LIVING SPACES IN BOTH HOLISTIC AND FENG SHUI DESIGN IS HIGHLY COMPATIBLE WITH THE NEEDS OF A WHEELCHAIR OR MOBILITY-AID USER. THERE IS ALSO NO REASON WHY FENG SHUI CANNOT BE USED TO IMPROVE THE PLACEMENT OF FURNITURE TO CREATE A MORE HARMONIOUS ATMOSPHERE. WOODEN OR LINOLEUM FLOORING MAY PROVIDE LESS RESISTANCE THAN CARPET AND MAKE GETTING AROUND EASIER, BUT FLOOR RUGS COULD BE A HINDRANCE OR EVEN DANGEROUS. THE FIELD OF VISION OF A PERSON IN A WHEELCHAIR, LIKE THAT OF A SMALL CHILD'S, NEEDS TO BE TAKEN INTO CONSIDERATION AND OBJECTS OF INTEREST SHOULD BE PLACED LOWER.

◆ FOR PEOPLE WITH BEHAVIORAL OR MENTAL HEALTH PROBLEMS—USE COLOR FOR ITS POSITIVE EMOTIONAL EFFECTS. A WARM SHADE OF BLUE IS VERY RELAXING FOR A CHILD WITH ATTENTION DEFICIT DISORDER, INDIGO IS SUCCESSFULLY USED BY COLOR THERAPISTS TO HELP THOSE WITH MENTAL HEALTH PROBLEMS; AND PINK HAS A SEDATING EFFECT TO COUNTER EMOTIONAL OUTBURSTS. FOR EVERY POSITIVE EFFECT, THERE ARE NEGATIVES ONES. RED, FOR EXAMPLE, IS VERY DISTURBING FOR A PERSON WITH A MENTAL HEALTH PROBLEM.

◆ SENSORY EXPERIENCES SHOULD NOT BE LIMITED TO THE HOUSE BUT THEY SHOULD SPRAWL INTO THE GARDEN AND WINDOW BOX. PLANTS—TENDING THEM, LOOKING AT THEM, INHALING THEIR SCENTS, HEARING THEM RUSTLE IN THE BREEZE, AND FEELING THEIR MYRIAD TEXTURES—ARE SENSORY THEME PARKS, OPEN TO EVERYONE.

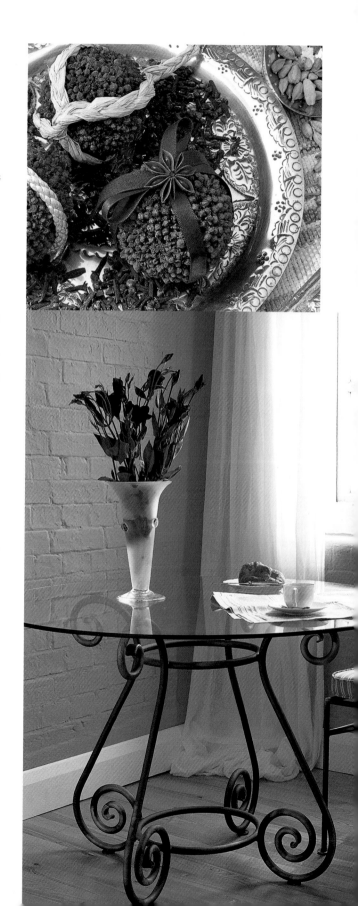

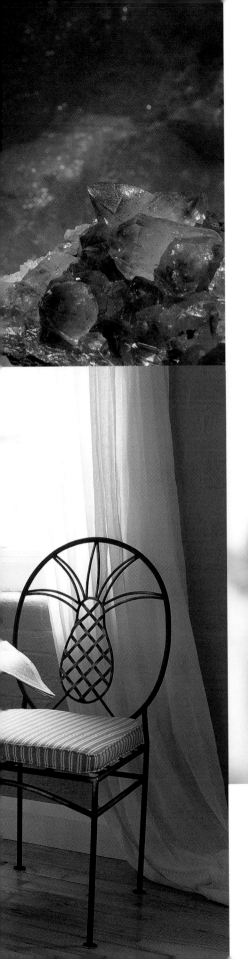

## Regal purples

Associated with the psychic and with intuition, purples are calming and soothing—they can create the right atmosphere for meditation. Purple is a royal color and as such is associated with wisdom and dignity, but it is also used in some cultures to symbolize sickness.

Indigo combines reason with intuition and discipline, and is associated with the process of change and the healing crisis.

It is seen by color therapists as cooling and astringent, and also as having an effect on vision, hearing, and smell. Indigo can be linked to stagnation, mental fatigue, and striving without success.

*Pomanders (FAR LEFT) were once carried to ward off sickness, so a purple binding is most appropriate.*

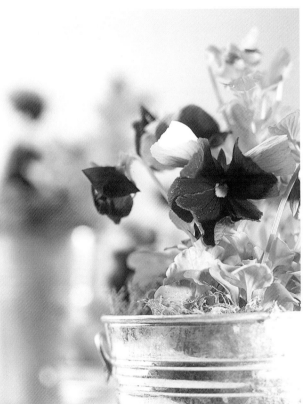

*A single flower, a shard of crystal (LEFT AND ABOVE), show purple in its most intense and most elusive shades.*

Violet is associated with good motives, spiritual aspirations, and prosperity. Color therapists say it is calming in mental illness, reduces hunger, and controls irritability. However, its negative associations include over-opulence, snobbery, and prejudice.

*Surround yourself with shades and hues of purple for a meditative mood (FAR LEFT).*

# 3air, light,

### s m e l l

Air, light, and smell are inextricably related, each affected by the quality and quantity of the other. There are many situations that can bring on the downward spiraling cycle of poor ventilation, insufficient natural light, and a stale atmosphere. But the important rule to remember and implement is that a healthy home needs lots of fresh air and natural light. These two alone are sufficient, but for atmosphere and for inspiration, the air should be filled with heavenly natural scents.

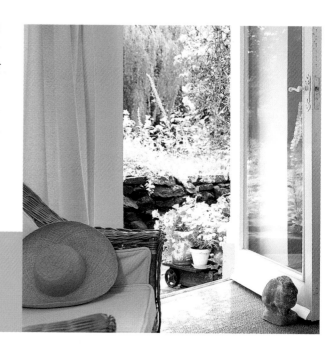

*"Smells are surer than sights and sounds to make the heart-strings crack."*

R U D Y A R D   K I P L I N G

While opening windows to get cross-ventilation, and airing rooms and furnishings seems simple enough, judging the effectiveness of your ventilation maneuvers can be difficult. What you need to do is sharpen your olfactory and tactile senses. To do this shut your eyes, therefore shutting down dominant visual feedback, and then take a walk around each room. Concentrate on smelling and feeling—locate where fresh air or even drafts are entering the room; where natural light strikes and warms your skin, a window sill or other surface; and where stale smells or cold air accumulate. Hopefully, you will also wander into pockets of air filled with the scent of cut flowers, candles, potpourris, and plants.

## AIR

Our relationship with air could not be more intimate. It moves in and out of our bodies every moment of our lives, and our planet's very existence relies upon it. The composition of air—78 percent nitrogen, 21 percent oxygen, and minute quantities of other gases—has remained stable for millions of years and is exactly right for maintaining life. Just a few more percent of either nitrogen or oxygen would threaten life on this planet.

The quality of the air we breathe affects us on every level. Fresh, clean air is not only health-giving, but also uplifting and inspirational, whereas polluted air fogs our brains, and wears down our health and spirit.

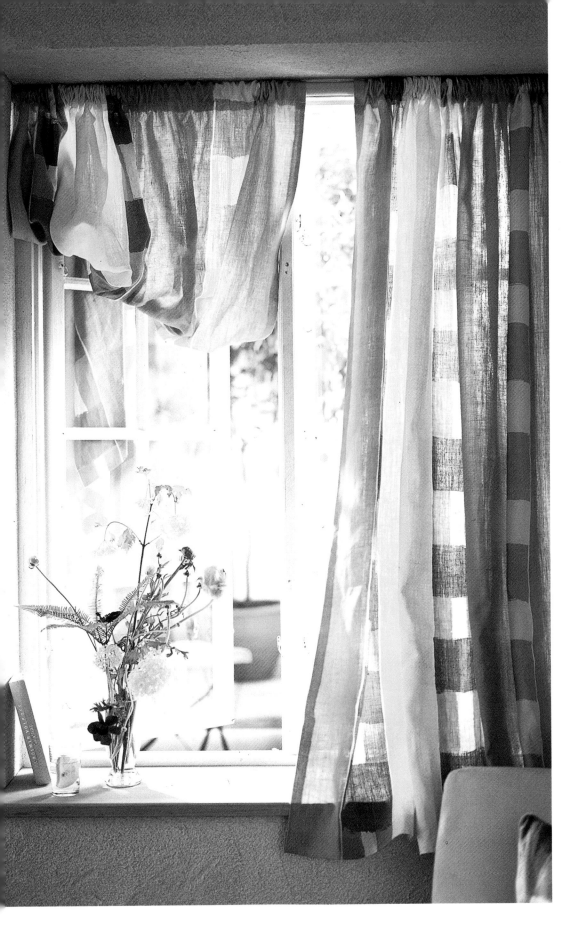

*F*resh air, natural light, and floral scents wafting through the home *(LEFT AND FAR LEFT) is health-* giving, uplifting, and cleansing.

## Air pollution—stifling health and spirit

Air-borne pollution knows no boundaries—mountain tops are capped in lead and car exhaust-saturated snow, cities choke on a cocktail of sulfur dioxide, carbon monoxide, nitrogen oxides, and lead; and even your home is an unwitting host to air pollution.

Synthetic building materials and furnishings, and chemical-based household products all emit toxic fumes that mix with dust, bacteria and fungi to sully air quality. Moreover, many homes are sealed to prevent drafts, or to allow artificial ventilation systems such as air conditioning to work, therefore stagnating the air even more. The home is further suffocated by the products we use to decorate and protect surfaces. Conventional paints, for example, prevent naturally-porous plaster or timber from breathing, and from releasing and absorbing moisture.

Equally important for our well-being is a balance between the positively charged protons and negatively charged electrons that make up the nuclei of molecules of air. Pollution causes negative electrons to be displaced, creating an excess of positive ions. Too many positive ions causes us to feel irritable, tense, and depressed. However, a surplus of negative ions appears to be beneficial. Interestingly, there are high concentrations of negative ions by the sea, in pine forests, and by waterfalls, which goes some way toward explaining their rejuvenating effects on our mood and health!

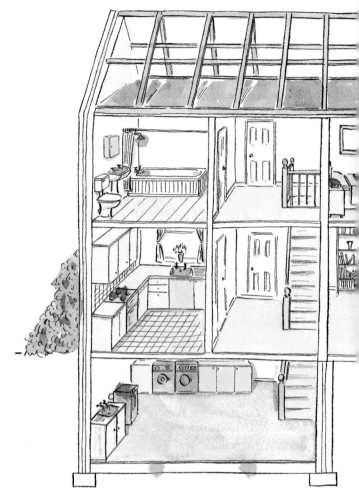

## Improving air quality in the home

You can assess the level of air pollution at home by taking stock of your health and that of your family. If anyone suffers regularly from headaches, itchy or watering eyes, nose or throat infections, dizziness, nausea, colds, asthma, or bronchitis, these may indicate air pollution. It may be found that symptoms are exacerbated when the home is tightly sealed during winter, or when the weather is hot and humid. You should also monitor if symptoms disappear when you leave the home, or if they are aggravated by certain events like spring cleaning, or products like paint or floor polishes.

The first step toward improving air quality is to remove or reduce sources of pollutants from the home. (See Detoxifying your home, page 14.)

The second step is to increase natural ventilation by regularly opening windows and doors, and using air vents and ducts. Air will then move naturally through the home due to pressure and temperature differences. Using extractor fans near sources of pollution can also help. Increasing air movement will make you feel fresher and more awake.

In older homes with fewer treated surfaces and less draft exclusion, air in the home would be exchanged every 60 minutes. But in modern homes with effective door and window seals, coated surfaces, and insulation, the process can take up to six hours.

It is also important to maintain comfortable humidity levels, particularly where heating systems dry the air. Humidifiers will do the job, but it is also worth thinking about hanging china

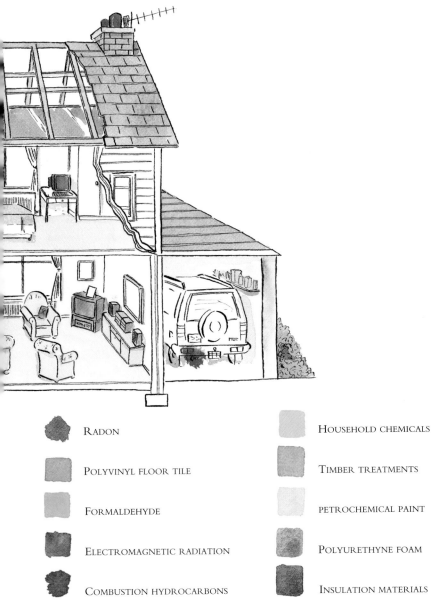

| | | | |
|---|---|---|---|
| ● | RADON | ● | HOUSEHOLD CHEMICALS |
| ● | POLYVINYL FLOOR TILE | ● | TIMBER TREATMENTS |
| ● | FORMALDEHYDE | ● | PETROCHEMICAL PAINT |
| ● | ELECTROMAGNETIC RADIATION | ● | POLYURETHYNE FOAM |
| ● | COMBUSTION HYDROCARBONS | ● | INSULATION MATERIALS |

# OFF-THE-SHELF *help*

✦ ELECTRONIC, FIBER OR CHARCOAL FILTERS—THESE REMOVE SOME POLLUTANTS, ALTHOUGH THEY DO NOT CLEAR TOXIC GASES. IRONICALLY, THEY CAN ALSO PROVIDE A NEW BREEDING GROUND FOR MOLDS IF THEY ARE NOT WELL-MAINTAINED.

✦ EXTRACTOR FANS—SUCK POLLUTED OR HUMID AIR AND VENT IT OUTSIDE. MANY HAVE REPLACEABLE FILTERS. PROPERLY MAINTAINED, THEY CAN BE EFFICIENT, IF NOISY. IN BATHROOMS WITHOUT WINDOWS, AN EXTRACTOR FAN IS OFTEN THE ONLY OPTION.

✦ HUMIDIFIERS—A RESERVOIR OF WATER INSIDE THE MACHINE IS SLOWLY HEATED TO BOILING POINT. THE STEAM IS THEN VENTED INTO THE ROOM. SOME BASIC MODELS ARE PORTABLE, WHILE SOPHISTICATED ONES COMBINE AIR PURIFYING AND HUMIDIFIER FUNCTIONS.

✦ IONIZERS—THESE CREATE AN ENVIRONMENT RICH IN NEGATIVE IONS, BY REMOVING SMOKE, DUST, AND SOME ALLERGENS FROM THE AIR. AN IONIZER HAS NO EFFECT ON TOXIC GASES, AND IT CAN BE DIFFICULT TO REMOVE MARKS ON NEARBY WALLS. MANY USERS REPORT A SIGNIFICANT IMPROVEMENT IN WELL-BEING.

✦ OZONE GENERATORS—SLIGHTLY CONTROVERSIAL BUT THEY AIM TO NEUTRALIZE TOXIC GASES, KILL BACTERIA AND MOLDS, AND DESTROY UNPLEASANT SMELLS.

water holders from radiators and having bowls of water placed around the home. Easier and more attractive solutions are: a vase of flowers, a bowl of petals or candles floating on water, an indoor water feature, or an aquarium. And while the original thinking behind the bedside jug of water and glass was to avoid a chilly, midnight walk to a cold kitchen, this simple gesture in a modern bedroom will humidify the air.

To rid air of pernicious vapors and chemicals, and at the same time improve humidity levels, overall air quality, and to add scent, look no further than plants. Some of the best are: spider plants, peace lilies, peperomia, dwarf banana plants, and mother-in-law's tongue.

*Modern homes, even more so than older ones, produce their own air pollution (ABOVE).*

## LIGHT

Without light, in the form of radiation from the Sun, there would be no life on Earth. All living things have evolved to follow the cycles of light and dark that occur as the Earth moves around the Sun. Circadian rhythms and our inner biological clock are tied in to these cycles. As the hours of sunlight shorten during winter months, we can become depressed and sluggish. Some people even suffer from seasonal affective disorder (SAD) because their exposure to sunlight is too limited.

"Light" in the form of the Sun has come to have many meanings in human society, and cultures have variously used it to symbolize wisdom, activity, and growth. Many cultures have worshiped the Sun, and we still recognize its potency in our language: "I saw the light," and "You are the light of my life."

### Natural light

Hour after hour, season by season, and from place to place, natural light is constantly changing. Early morning fall light, slightly clouded by mist, is very different to the early evening light of a cloudless summer's day; and the harsh light of the tropics bears little resemblance to its more subtle equivalent in northern America or Europe.

The quality of light coming into your home also varies. It can be direct, reflected off other surfaces before it arrives, or diffused through drapes, blinds or textured glass. The color and strength of the light will also depend on the materials it bounces off or penetrates. A stain glass window, or lead crystals or prisms hung in a window, will flood a room with a rainbow of colors.

The function of a room should determine the quality and quantity of light needed. Kitchens, work rooms, and playrooms benefit from plenty of direct sunlight, whereas a living room, bedroom, meditation area or bathroom will feel more relaxed with reflected or diffused lighting. Lighting in an entranceway or hallway should be flexible so as to meet practical requirements and to create a welcoming atmosphere at all times. During the day it should be flooded with warm natural light, while at a night a creative combination of artificial light and candles can be used.

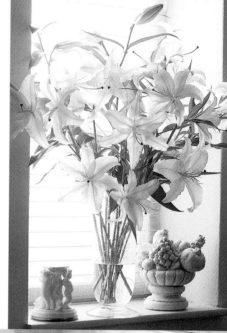

*More than simply scented decoration, fresh flowers (RIGHT) can improve air quality in your home.*

*Lower the need for blanket artificial lighting and add atmosphere with candles (BELOW).*

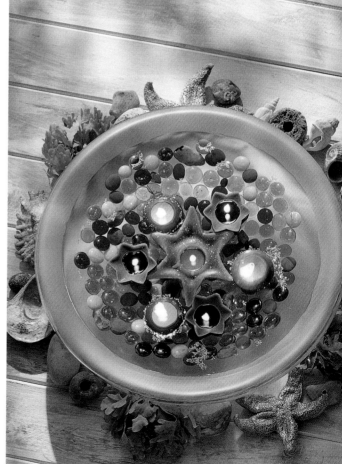

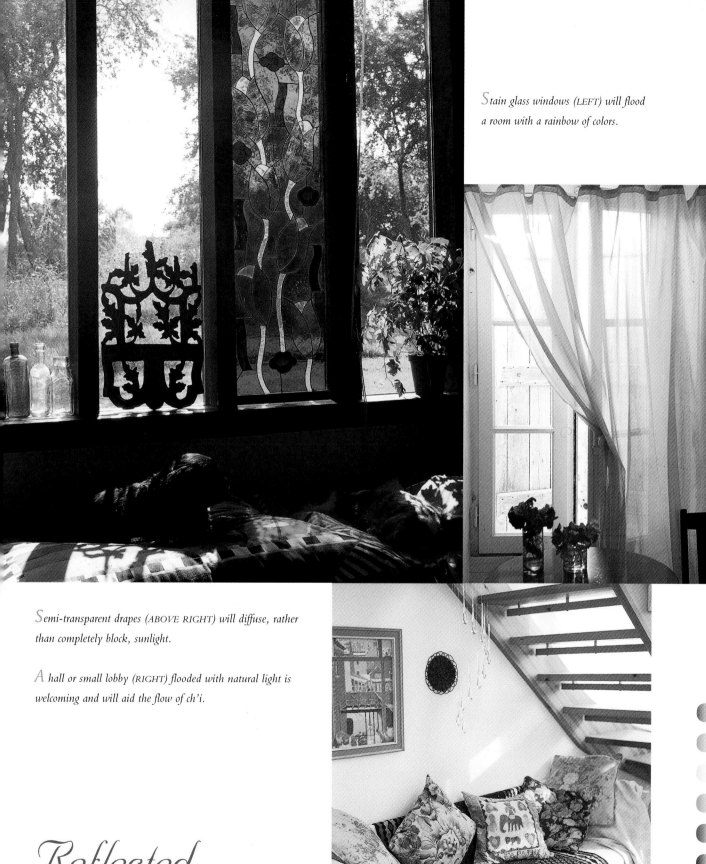

*S*tain glass windows (LEFT) will flood a room with a rainbow of colors.

*S*emi-transparent drapes (ABOVE RIGHT) will diffuse, rather than completely block, sunlight.

*A* hall or small lobby (RIGHT) flooded with natural light is welcoming and will aid the flow of ch'i.

*Reflected*

DIFFUSED

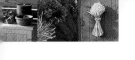

# CANDLE
*magic*

*A*ccording to traditional lore, candles of certain colors have different symbolic meanings.

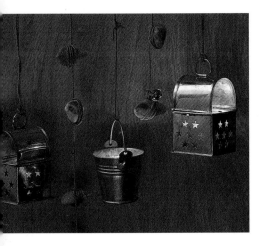

*A* gently glowing column of soft light—the perfect artificial lighting solution for a bedroom (*RIGHT*).

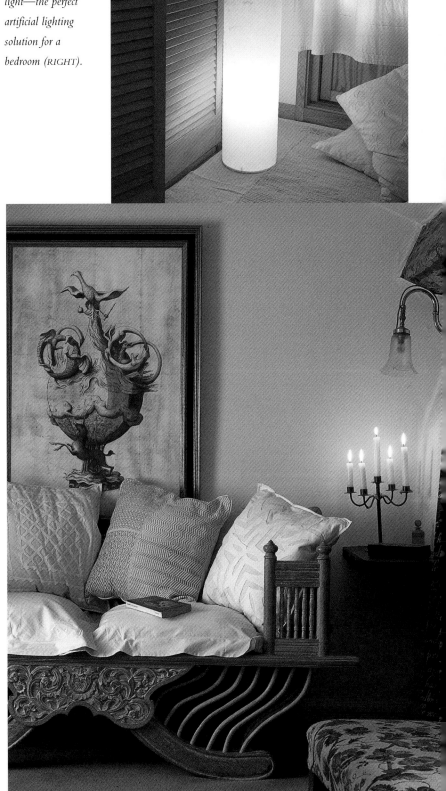

✦ WHITE CANDLES FOR PEACE AND SPIRITUALITY; RED TO PROTECT THE HOME AND THOSE IN IT; HEALING ENERGIES, LUCK, AND PROSPERITY ARE DERIVED FROM GREEN CANDLES; AND YELLOW CREATES THE RIGHT MOOD FOR STUDY OR READING. PINK CANDLES GENERATE FRIENDSHIP AND LOVING FEELINGS, MAKING PINK THE PERFECT CHOICE FOR PARTIES AND ROMANTIC DINNERS. PURPLE SPEEDS HEALING, AND A BLUE CANDLE WILL PROTECT YOU WHILE YOU SLEEP. PROBLEM SOLVING IS BEST DONE UNDER THE FLICKER OF A BROWN CANDLE.

*B*urning white candles (*RIGHT*) is believed to bring peace and spirituality to a room. Creative use of artificial lighting (*FAR RIGHT*) to highlight a decorative feature.

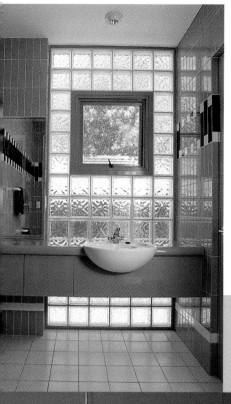

*A glass brick wall, with inset window, (LEFT) maximizes natural light and ventilation in a bathroom.*

## Maximizing natural light

You can maximize the amount of natural light entering your home by cutting back shrubs, bushes, and trees that are blocking light, by keeping windows clean, and by drawing window dressings back to expose the whole window. An easy remedy is to hang mirrors so that they bounce light into recesses or dark corners. Sunlight-starved rooms will benefit from light-colored paints, wallpapers, and furnishings.

When planning an extension, or any structural changes to your home, the location of windows should be given careful consideration so that you can extend natural lighting possibilities. Adding a skylight—even a small one—or a window facing in a direction different to those already in place, for example, will transform a room.

*"And Life is Colour and Warmth and Light"*

J U L I A N   G R E N F E L L

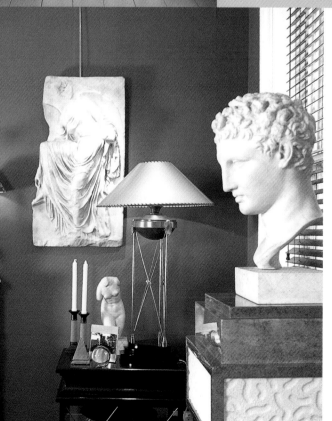

## Artificial light

Most of us rely on electric lighting, but we often fail to make the best use of it. Used creatively and sensitively it will reflect your mood and add atmosphere; used incorrectly it can affect your health. Fluorescent bulbs, for example, can increase feelings of irritability and fatigue, and are implicated in allergies and attention deficit disorder. The aim should be to make artificial lighting as "natural" as possible. One way of doing this is by using full-spectrum lamps, which have bulbs that replicate the spectral balance of daylight, and emit slightly higher levels of ultraviolet than ordinary bulbs.

Overhead, central lighting is most common, but sadly also the least creative. Much better to have a flexible lighting system consisting of varied light sources: downlights, uplights, spotlights, table lamps, and floor lamps. Install a dimmer switch so that even overhead lighting can be set to meet your mood and needs.

Atmospheric alternatives to electric lighting—kerosene (paraffin) or oil lamps, and candles—offer a soft, glowing light that is almost mystical.

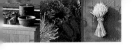

### FENG SHUI AND LIGHTING

Light—natural and artificial—helps to activate ch'i energy. Uplights will promote ch'i to flow up so that it moves onto upper floors and galleries, or into the upper reaches of unusually steep or pitched ceilings. Spotlights, low-voltage lighting, lamps, and candles will increase the flow of ch'i through stagnant areas.

Bare light bulbs or very harsh lighting are very yang. Balance this by introducing yin using lampshades, paper screens or even plants to soften the light.

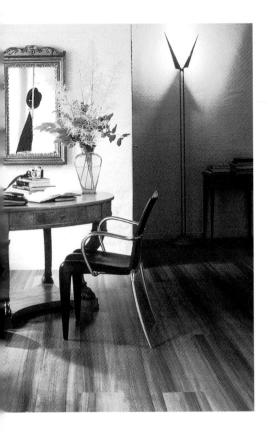

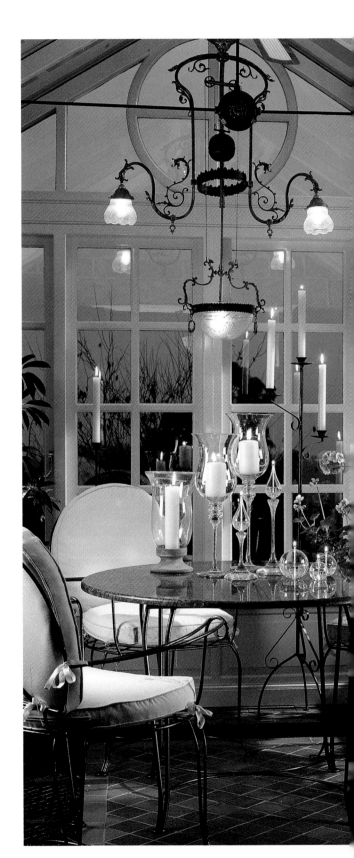

*Lights can be used to increase the flow of ch'i in stagnant corners (LEFT).*

Candles bring fire ch'i energy into a room, which the Chinese believe encourages passion and expressiveness. White candles are preferred because they have the greatest affinity to the actual flame. Candle holders also play their part in influencing ch'i. This belief stems from the relationship between certain materials and ch'i energies in the Five Elements (page 17). A tall, black wrought-iron candle holder is associated with tree, soil, and metal energies, whereas a flat, white china holder is linked to soil energy.

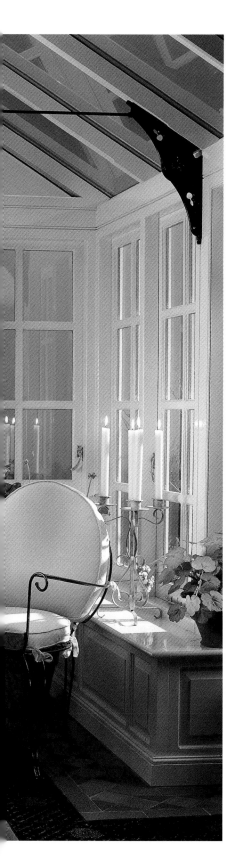

## SMELL

Whether it is the heady aroma of honeysuckle, the smell of baking bread, or the milky scent of a baby, smells affect us. Our sense of smell is a powerful one, so powerful that we can recall smells years after experiencing them only once and for a short period. Receptors in our nose can detect a single molecule of a scent, and our bodies will react to a smell even if we are not actually conscious of it.

Different smells will conjure different emotions, memories, and associations for each of us, and the smells in our home will therefore affect how we feel about it. Research suggests that smells can affect our energy levels, and aromatherapists have been using strong-smelling essential oils in their healing arts for years. Vanilla and sandalwood essential oils are said to calm nerves, while geranium, bergamot, and rosemary will lift the spirits. Relaxation is promised by lavender, ylang ylang, and neroli essential oils.

Not all smells are pleasant, or health-giving. Every day we are bombarded with tobacco smoke, traffic exhaust fumes, synthetic air fresheners and polishes, and so on—and these are only a few of the ones we consciously detect. There are thousands more that can damage our health, yet pass unnoticed.

*A magical atmosphere (LEFT) created by candles and the scent of beeswax and essential oils.*

*A screen of flourishing plants (BELOW) diffuse light and release their scent.*

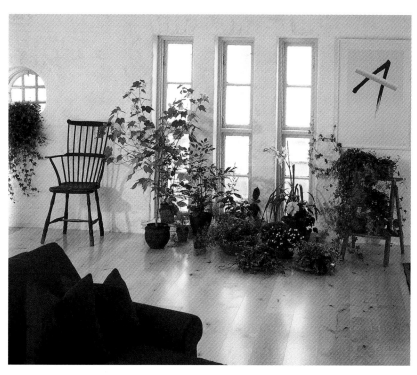

### Creating a fragrant home

Every home has its own characteristic smell, but it can be altered by cleansing the air with spray mists, by bringing sweet-smelling, fresh flowers into a room, or by growing aromatic herbs and plants on window sills or wherever they will thrive. Lemon verbena, lilies, jasmine, and violets, for example, all have lovely scents that will intensify in warm conditions and be released every time they are brushed against or caught in a breeze.

Natural materials also come with their own earthy and sensual odors. There are the unmistakable smells of a camphor chest, bamboo blinds, sisal matting, and, of course, natural-scented furniture polish.

Lighting incense burners is believed both to honor the divine and to clear a house of negative energy. Each scent has different powers and influence. Those associated with health and healing include cedar, cinnamon, myrrh, rose, sandalwood, and gardenia. Incense ingredients are available ready-ground or in blocks.

Heighten the potency of essential oils by mixing a few drops of oil with a little water, and heating it over a flame in special burner. The heat from the candle warms the water, liberating the scent into the room.

# SCENTED MAGIC
*in the air*

*A*s smell is a very personal thing, each of us must select the smells *we like. Here are just a few recipes to choose from.*

### Refreshing potpourri

In a sealable glass container or polythene bag, mix together 2 oz fresh lemon verbena leaves; 3 oz fresh lavender flowers; 1 oz fresh peppermint leaves; 1 oz fresh marjoram leaves; a selection of blue or mauve petals for decoration; ½ nutmeg (grated); 1 tablespoon blade mace (crushed); 1 oz orris root powder; and 1 drop each of lavender, lemon, orange blossom, and peppermint essential oils. Seal the container or bag, and store in a cool, dry place for six weeks. Shake the mixture daily. When ready, decant into a ceramic or wooden bowl.

### Incense for health

Grind and mix together the following ingredients: two parts myrrh, two parts sandalwood, one part sage, and one part rosemary. Burn the incense in an earthenware or ceramic bowl when someone in the home is unwell.

### Herb pillows

Combine two or three of your favorite dried herbs with a few drops of rosemary or oregano essential oil in a bowl. Mix together thoroughly. Fill small muslin or cheesecloth pillows with a spoonful or two of the herb concoction.

### Clove pomanders

Gently knead an orange to soften the skin. Stick cloves all over the orange, leaving a space between each to allow for shrinkage. To make a hanging pomander, leave room for a narrow ribbon to be wound around the orange. Mix one tablespoon of orris root power with one tablespoon of ground cinnamon, and roll the orange in it. Make sure the pomander is well coated before wrapping it in tissue. Store in a paper bag in a dark, airy place for two to three weeks.

### Homemade furniture polish:

Mix ½ cup of both linseed oil and malt vinegar in a glass jar. Add 40 crushed sweet cicely seeds, or 1½ teaspoons of lavender essential oil and four drops of peppermint essential oil. If cicely seeds are used, the mixture should be left in a warm place for two weeks and shaken daily. If essential oils are used, the polish can be used immediately.

### Zesty air freshener

Barely fill a ½ cup spray mist bottle with purified water and add the following essential oils: 50 drops each of lime and grapefruit, and 10 drops each of orange and patchouli. Shake well and spray the mist into the air.

### Carpet freshener

Mix the following oils in a jar containing ½ cup baking soda: 60 drops lavender, and 20 drops each of cinnamon and orange. Seal the jar and leave for 24 hours. Sprinkle onto the carpet, leave for 15 minutes and then vacuum.

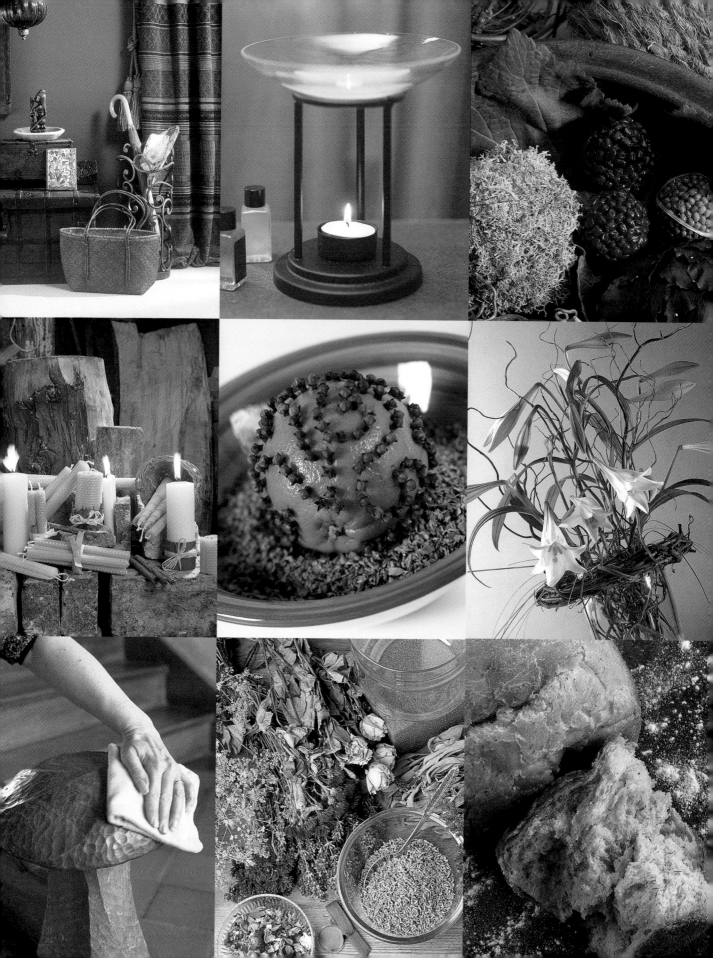

# 4 sound

Sound touches our minds, bodies and spirits. Beautiful music can inspire, the sound of nature soothe, and noise pollution send our stress levels soaring.

Unlike the senses of sight and smell, which rely on specific receptors, all the cells in our body respond to sound, even if the sound is below the level of conscious awareness. So sounds never cease to have an effect. According to Native American Indian culture, every animal and plant has its own sound vibration, and "silent sound" is used to call animals to the hunt and to find plants.

In many traditional cultures, sound is used to cleanse and clear the energy in a home and to create a harmonious atmosphere. Any musical instrument can be used—in some cultures pots and pans are banged to get rid of evil spirits or "bad energy;" in others drums are beaten or bells rung.

## NOISE

Most of us underestimate the negative effects of sound, although noise is now recognized as a health hazard, and noise abatement laws exist in many countries.

Whether at work, out shopping, or at home, we are all bombarded with noise. Traffic, construction work, airplanes, dogs barking, household appliances, and office equipment, and so on can all disturb our peace. The loudness, or intensity, of some noises are actually dangerous. The noise produced by a food blender is only 20 decibels (a decibel is the unit used to measure the loudness of sound) below the threshold of pain; and the shrill of an alarm clock, at 80 decibels, is on the danger level. Washing machines and vacuum cleaners are a little better, but not much.

> *"The man that hath no music in himself,*
> *Nor is not mov'd with concord of sweet sounds,*
> *Is fit for treasons, stratagems, and spoils;*
> *The motions of his spirit are dull as night…*
>
> "THE MERCHANT OF VENICE"
> WILLIAM SHAKESPEARE

*The benefit of an indoor water feature (RIGHT) goes beyond its value as decorative feature. The sound of water bubbling over stones and the tinkling of a fountain are relaxing and will stimulate ch'i. And just as a natural waterfall encourages beneficial negative ion concentrations, moving water in the home can do the same, albeit on a much smaller scale.*

## *Inspire, cleanse*
### SOOTHE, CLEAR

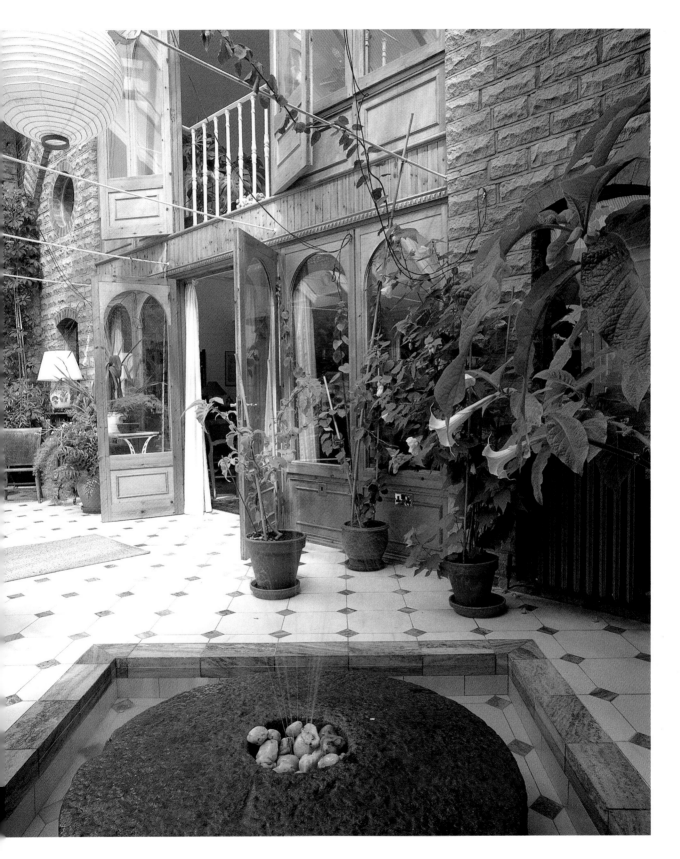

S
O
U
N
D

### Silencing the racket

✦ Plant a barrier of trees, or construct a mound of soil and rocks that will absorb or deflect noise. Turn this natural sound barrier into a rock or alpine garden, or you can opt for an ascetic Japanese look. Fences and walls will be more effective if planted up with a hedge, or covered with creepers. Internal or external wooden shutters, secondary glazing on windows, and extra-heavy drapes will also keep intrusive noise at bay.

✦ Put kitchen appliances on rubber mats and position them away from partition walls. Rubber mats, wooden boards, and coil mats set under pots and pans will muffle the bangs and crashes associated with food preparation.

✦ Partition walls, or common walls, can be made more soundproof by placing bookshelves against them. When filled with books, you reduce external noise intrusion, and also deaden noise within the room.

✦ To make a room quieter, fill it with lots of "absorbent" surfaces. Pile cushions and throws or decorative blankets onto sofas and chairs, hang rugs on walls, and even scatter rugs over carpeted flooring.

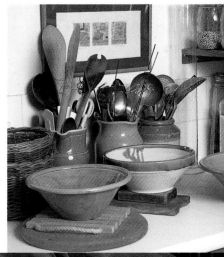

*Wooden boards under pots and bowls (RIGHT) will reduce the noises associated with cooking.*

*Book-lined shelves (LEFT) are an attractive and practical method of sound-proofing.*

*An exotic but very quiet bedroom, (RIGHT) thanks to heavy drapes, cushions, carpet, and a canopy*

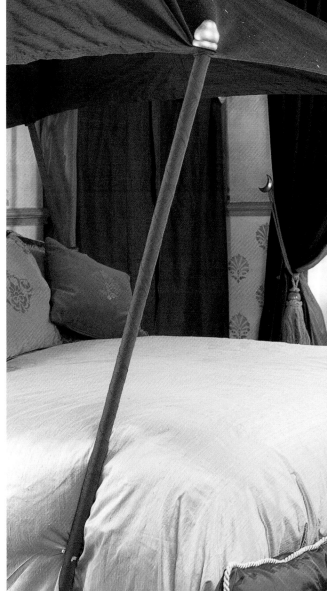

50

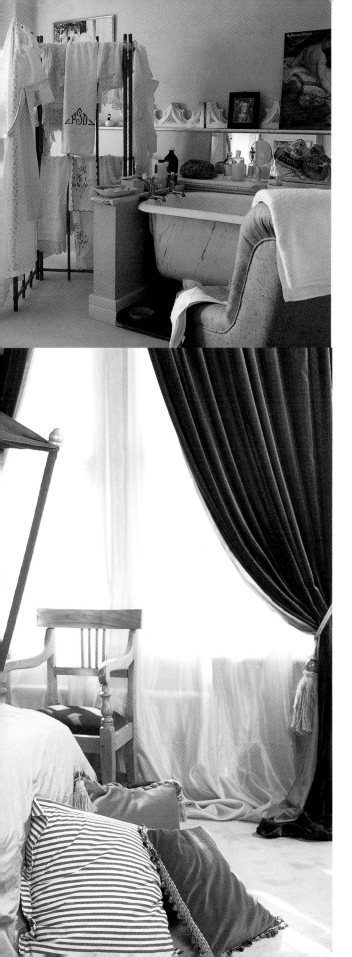

◆ Homes are full of incidental noises—the ring of the telephone, the buzz of a doorbell, alarms, slamming doors, creaking floorboards—that jar, grate, and set your nerves on edge, but nothing is ever done about them. There are quiet solutions to these problems—some easy, and some not so easy, as anyone with creaking floorboards will attest. You can turn down the bell on a phone, and replace a door buzzer with a brass knocker or pull-chain bell. A shrill, wake-the-dead alarm clock should be placed on a rubber mat and covered with a heavy cloth, or you can mute the hammer by winding tape around it. And say goodbye to slamming doors by fitting good, old-fashioned door stops.

*Rails (LEFT) or shelves of towels will reduce noisy reverberation in a bathroom, as will introducing Japanese-style wooden floor mats (RIGHT).*

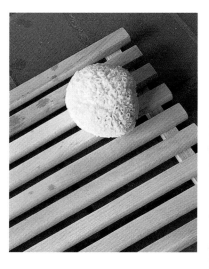

◆ Sparsely decorated, and with tile walls and tile flooring, a bathroom can be a very noisy room. Warm up the atmosphere and soften the sound by bringing in plants, and laying washable rugs or Japanese-style wooden mats on the floor. Stifle noisy plumbing with shelves of towels, and consider installing a silent flush toilet. Replace plastic and nylon items—laundry basket, shower screens and curtains—with natural, sound-absorbing raffia, wood, and cotton fabrics.

◆ Introduce a few home rules to lower the decibel level. You could restrict the use of noisy appliances to specific times so that evenings are peaceful, and go barefoot or wear soft-soled shoes indoors. If the background noise level is lowered, then many other activities will also be carried out at lower volume.

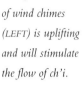

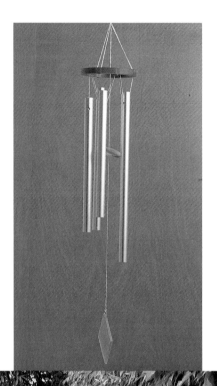

*The gentle tinkle of wind chimes (LEFT) is uplifting and will stimulate the flow of ch'i.*

*A hedge and climbing creeper as a buffer against suburban noise; bamboo to create desired natural music (BELOW).*

## FENG SHUI AND SOUND

Sound vibrations stimulate ch'i energy. You can improve your personal ch'i by chanting and singing, and that of your home by using wind chimes, a burbling water feature, bells, and gongs. Even the patient and regular ticking and chiming of an old grandfather clock can generate an ordered ch'i that will bring calm to the most chaotic household.

Use wind chimes inside and outside the home. The sweeter and clearer their sound, the better they will purify and cleanse ch'i energy. Chimes can be made from metal, wood or pottery, but it is important to choose the right material for the place you wish to set your chimes. To stimulate ch'i energy near a door in the north of a home, for example, chimes need to be of metal and hung so that they catch the movement of air as a door is opened or closed.

A water feature does not have to be a fountain on a grand scale. A simple and inexpensive pump and water-recycling system can be installed in a clay, concrete, galvanised metal or wooden container, into the earth face of a grotto, or set to run over a pile of pebbles. The compact pumps now available mean that it is quite easy to create an imaginative indoor water feature.

Bells and gongs are used to clear ch'i energy that has become stagnant. And the tools to correct that stagnant ch'i are at your fingertips in the form of a metal door knocker or sweet-sounding doorbell.

### Creating the sounds you want

Once you have tackled noise pollution, you can start to use sound positively, for enjoyment and relaxation. There are many beautiful sounds that you can introduce: wind chimes, a gently burbling water feature, or a tape of natural sound recordings that can bring a rainforest, or a school of dolphins into your home.

Not only can your garden protect you from unwanted noises, it can be the source of delightful natural music. Reeds, poplars, and bamboo will rustle in the wind, and there can be bird-song aplenty if you encourage them into your garden with berry-producing shrubs .

# 5 energy
## EFFICIENCY

We use a great deal of energy and pay a premium for the conveniences it offers; we also waste a great deal. The combination of energy avarice and inefficiency has an enormous impact on the environment, causing acid rain, and contributing to the greenhouse effect. But with simple energy conservation measures, it is possible to reduce substantially the amount of energy we use and lose, and at the same time make our homes and our lives more holistic.

### Energy guzzlers

Maintaining our homes so that they are warm in winter and cool in summer constitutes our greatest energy inefficiencies. There is the tendency to wind up the controls so that we either bake or freeze. Correcting these extremes is then usually done by opening or closing doors and windows so that expensively heated or cooled air is vented outside. Other options, even the obvious one of carefully adjusting the appliance's temperature setting and timer, are often neglected in the pursuit of immediate comfort.

Flick-of-a-switch convenience—hot water, ice-makers, washing machines and the rest—has improved the quality of life and our health profiles, but there is a downside.

Appliances, and heating and cooling systems are noisy or provide a background "hum" that we come to take for granted; they choke the air with electromagnetic radiation and toxic fumes; and they can be dangerous, but they also "sterilize" our lives. Why knead bread when the dough-maker can do it? Why put on a sweater when the heating can be turned up? Why do something by hand when there is a power gadget that will do it for you?

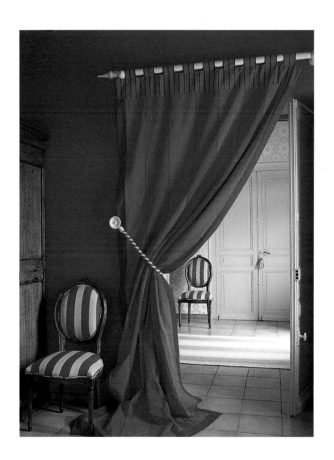

*Hanging heavy, lined drapes inside external or internal doors (ABOVE) will prevent drafts, form an air trap, and conserve heat.*

An holistic home is one that achieves a balance between convenience and energy conservation. To conserve energy, first look at the ways in which your home wastes it. Armed with that information you can then make effective changes to your use—or misuse—of it.

## Energy sources

Many of us have no choice about which energy sources have been utilized in our home, but when we do have a say, what are the arguments for and against each energy provider?

**Coal**  Some 90 percent of the heat from a coal fire vanishes up the chimney, so despite the cosy flames, coal fires are inefficient. Coal also emits many toxic gases, radioactive potassium-40 and carbon-14, and was responsible for the smogs of the past and the accompanying respiratory diseases.

**Electricity**  This is generated by water, or by burning coal and oil. Hydroelectric power destroys river and lake systems, while coal and oil—both non-renewable resources—cause water and air pollution.

**Natural gas**  This is mostly methane, which burns efficiently giving off only water vapor and carbon dioxide. Produced by the partial decomposition of living organisms that lived millions of years ago, it is non-renewable.

**Nuclear power**  The decay of radioactive fuel releases heat that turns water to steam. The steam drives turbines that are connected to generators. While controversy rages about the disposal of nuclear waste, nuclear power is— provided power stations meet stringent safety standards—safe and clean.

**Solar power**  Solar cells harness sunlight and use it to heat water that provides both hot water and heating. Solar panels on homes are popular in hot countries, but new technology is making them more efficient for use in less sunny climes.

**Wind, wave, and tidal power**  To match the output of a conventional power station, wind generators would have to cover huge areas of high land, wave generators would measure miles in length, and the barrages that would harness tidal power would have to be set across almost every available bay, inlet, and estuary. Even though these alternative power sources are non-polluting and use renewable resources, they would have negative effects on the environment. They will displace or upset the flora and fauna, and land, often scenic or of special interest, which is given over to noisy, wind-generating farms would be inaccessible to the public. The financial cost of providing and buying these alternative energies is about the same as conventional energy sources.

**Wood**  People seeking a more natural lifestyle often look no further than a beautiful wood-burning stove or Aga to provide heat, hot water, and a cooking oven. Yet, a wood-burning stove is one of the most polluting, emitting a dangerous cocktail of soot, water vapor, ash, carcinogenic hydrocarbons, carbon monoxide, sulfur dioxide, and carbon dioxide. Coal-burning stoves may be more efficient, but they too emit fumes of sulfur dioxide, carbon dioxide, and some hydrocarbons.

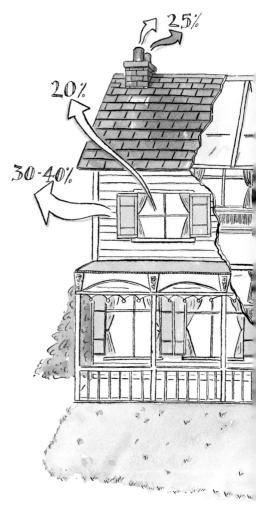

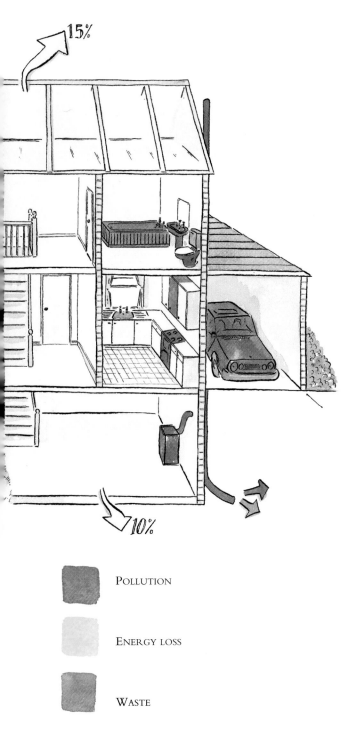

15%

10%

POLLUTION

ENERGY LOSS

WASTE

## HOW TO SAVE ENERGY

It may be that the best we can do, in light of what we know about energy sources, is to use as little energy as possible, and to make our homes as energy-efficient as possible.

### Heating

Some 25 percent of heat escapes through the roof, over 30 percent through non-insulated walls, and 16 percent through ground floors. Roof insulation is basically a do-it-yourself job, but wall and floor insulation should be undertaken by a qualified tradesman. Gaps in ground-floor floorboards or between flooring and wall can be filled with papier-mâché. When dry, sand the papier-mâché to a smooth finish.

Double glazing, secondary glazing, and adhesive insulation strips will cut heat loss through windows, as will fixing clear polythene sheeting directly to the glass surface. This material is shrunk to fit using the heat from a hair drier, and can be removed during the summer. Plug unused chimney flues with newspaper, and hang heavy, lined drapes inside external doors that are exposed to chill winds. Create an air-trap between external doors and adjoining areas with a retractable floor-to-ceiling screen or heavy drapes.

Some rooms need less heating than others. This is not only energy-efficient, but also beneficial for health and vitality. A home that is a consistent temperature throughout, induces lethargy. Bedrooms—even those of very young children or older people—and studies or dens require less heating, than living areas.

Turn down the thermostat or temperature setting on the hot water cylinder or boiler, and heating system. If you do it gradually over a few days, you will not even notice the difference. Insulate the cylinder and hot water pipes with lagging to prevent unnecessary heat loss.

Central heating radiators can be made more efficient by fitting a shelf directly above them. The shelf forces the heat to move out into the room rather than rise to the ceiling. Aluminum foil can also be taped behind radiators to reflect heat into the room and not through the walls.

*An average house loses an astounding amount of energy (LEFT), and conventional building technology has done little to remedy it.*

## Cooling

To reduce reliance on air-conditioning systems or electric fans, insulate roof and walls, or tape aluminum foil to the inside of the roof space to reduce heat absorption by up to 20 percent. Provide lots of ventilation so that cool air enters through lower windows or doors, forcing hot air out through upper storey windows or vents.

Install wide awnings over windows exposed to direct sun, or plant deciduous trees in front of those windows so that they block the sun and create a shady screen. Drapes or blinds lined with a reflective material will also help.

Maximize the cooling effect of an enclosed electric fan by hanging a wet sheet in front of it. When the sheet dries, soak it again. This is particularly effective when cooling a small room, or to create a more comfortable environment for very young babies or older people.

During especially hot spells, be flexible and practical. It is not uncommon in Australia, for example, for health practitioners to recommend that babies and young children sleep in the bathroom where it is cooler.

## Appliances

Buy energy-efficient appliances such as electric skillets and slow cookers as they use less energy than ovens and stoves, and prune your kitchen of energy-guzzling gadgets. It is now also possible to buy refrigerators, freezer cabinets, and washing machines that are energy-efficient. In some countries these appliances are being graded according to their energy-efficiency. An appliance with an A rating is environmentally very friendly and highly energy-efficient, and will reduce your energy bills. The lowest rating is G.

To improve the efficiency of stoves and ovens, keep heating plates and reflective surfaces clean. Make sure the lids of cooking pots and pans fit properly, and that pans cover a heating element completely. Boil only as much water as you need.

Open the refrigerator or freezer as infrequently as you can. Each time the door is opened, cold air escapes and extra power is used to reduce the internal temperature again. Do not leave televisions or video machines on remote control overnight. Switch them off properly.

*M*agenta red and burnished orange (RIGHT) create a cosy corner.

*W*ide awnings and louver shutters on doors and windows (BELOW) protect this home from the hottest rays of the sun.

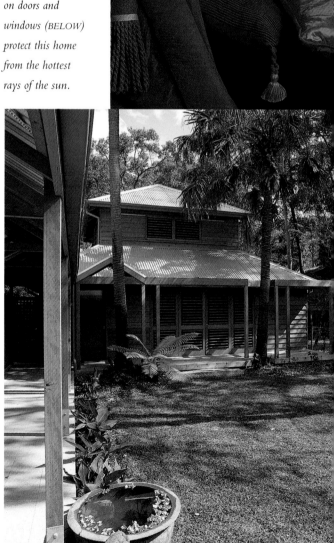

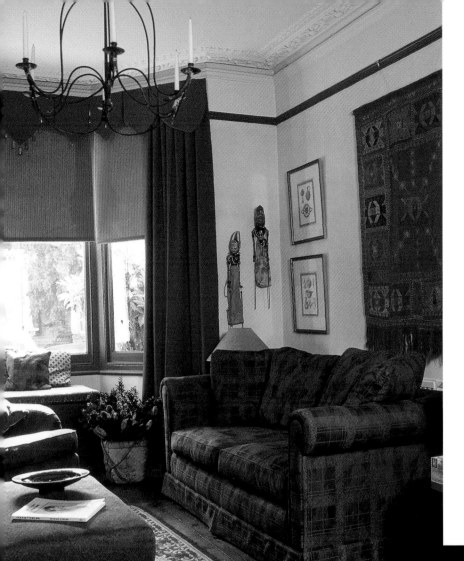

# FURNITURE
*and decoration*

*Y*ou can heighten feelings of warmth or
coolness by using appropriate colors,
and by rearranging furniture to suit the
season and climate.

✦ TO CREATE A COSY, WARM
FEELING, PILE TEXTURED CUSHIONS
ONTO SOFAS THAT ARE DRAPED
WITH COMFORTABLE THROWS,
RUGS, AND BLANKETS.

✦ ADJUST ARTIFICIAL LIGHTING TO
REDUCE THE SIZE OF A ROOM—A
LARGE ROOM ALWAYS SEEMS COLDER
THAN A SMALL ONE—AND TO FOCUS
ATTENTION ON INTERESTING DETAILS
WITHIN THE ROOM.

*A* living room (ABOVE) designed and
furnished for colder climes, using heavy
fabrics and rugs in a medley of warm colors.

*P*ockets of low lighting (RIGHT) are used to
make this large room appear much smaller
and therefore warmer.

CHAPTER

# 6 entrance
ENTRANCE

THE WAYS IN WHICH HOLISTIC DESIGN AND FENG SHUI CAN BE USED TO ENHANCE YOUR HOME AND LIFESTYLE ARE TOO NUMEROUS TO COVER IN JUST ONE BOOK. THEY BOTH REALLY DESERVE A LIFETIME OF STUDY AND PURSUIT. DIP INTO THIS SECTION AND USE THE IDEAS AND TIPS THAT YOU FEEL COMFORTABLE WITH, MIXING THEM TOGETHER TO CREATE A POTPOURRI OF INSPIRATION. THERE IS NOTHING TO BE GAINED FROM SLAVISHLY FOLLOWING A COLOR SUGGESTION, FOR EXAMPLE, IF YOU ABSOLUTELY CANNOT STAND THAT PARTICULAR COLOR. ON MOST ISSUES, HOLISTIC DESIGN AND FENG SHUI ARE IN ACCORD, BUT WHERE THERE IS CONFLICTING ADVICE, YOU MUST DECIDE WHICH BEST SATISFIES YOUR NEEDS. ALWAYS CHOOSE A PATH THAT REFLECTS YOUR PRIORITIES—HOLISM AND FENG SHUI WOULD NOT HAVE IT ANY OTHER WAY.

USE THE INFORMATION AND IDEAS IN THIS SECTION IN CONJUNCTION WITH THOSE IN THE SACRED HOME CHAPTER THAT DEAL IN MORE DETAIL WITH COLOR, LIGHT, AIR, SMELL, SOUND, AND ENERGY EFFICIENCY.

The front door is the threshold between the outside world and the internal world of the home. The path or porch, and hallway are the avenues that bring you to this threshold. In traditional lore, the front door was hung with charms or was the focus of rituals that would protect the home and its inhabitants from evil. But the entrance is not just about repeling unwanted influences: it is also an opportunity to invite positive energies into the home. Placing five shiny coins on the porch, for example, was thought to bless a home with love and prosperity. Auspicious energies will make your home more welcoming.

First and foremost is good lighting. An entrance should be flooded with natural light during the day, and filled with gentle, atmospheric lighting at night. If deprived of sunlight, a dark entrance hall is best illuminated by uplights. Their light, reflected off space-enhancing, pale-colored ceilings and walls, or mirrors, most closely approximates natural light.

The second consideration is color. Because an entrance area has two distinct functions—introducing a guest to your home, and providing a practical thoroughfare between rooms—the decoration has to be both warm and light. Rich and sumptuous reds may look warm and inviting at night, but oppressive and dark by day when the hall fulfills its functional role.

## Threshold
PROTECT

Both functions are best served if an entrance area is uncluttered, making it more inviting and encouraging the energy of the home to flow more harmoniously. Determine what are the area's most important functions, and provide furniture and decoration to meet only those needs.

The third consideration is giving the entrance area atmosphere. Color and lighting are certainly important in this, but do not overlook the impact of texture, sound, and smell. A noisy, echoing hall, for example, does not provide a welcoming ambience for anyone.

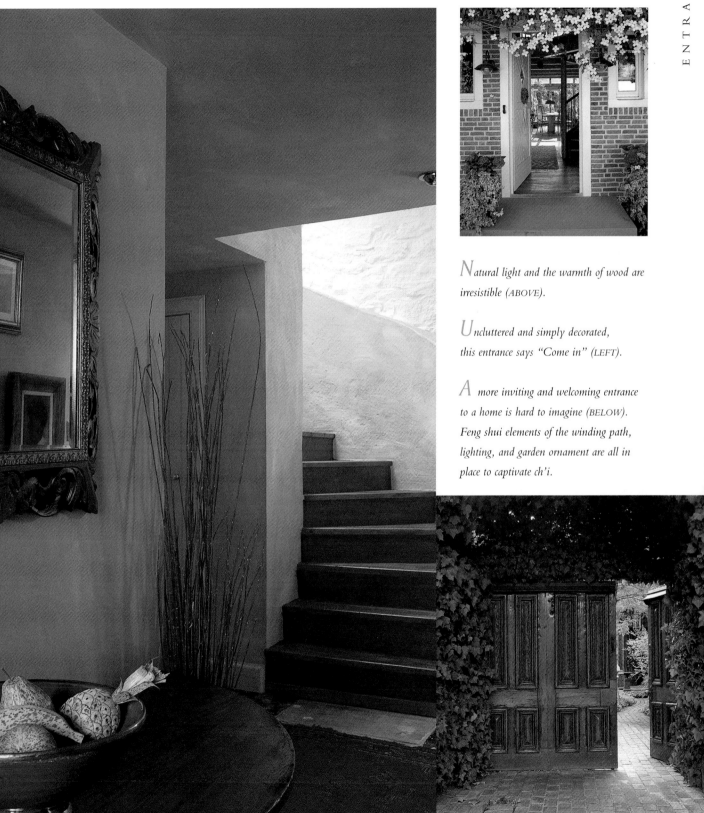

*N*atural light and the warmth of wood are irresistible (ABOVE).

*U*ncluttered and simply decorated, this entrance says "Come in" (LEFT).

*A* more inviting and welcoming entrance to a home is hard to imagine (BELOW). Feng shui elements of the winding path, lighting, and garden ornament are all in place to captivate ch'i.

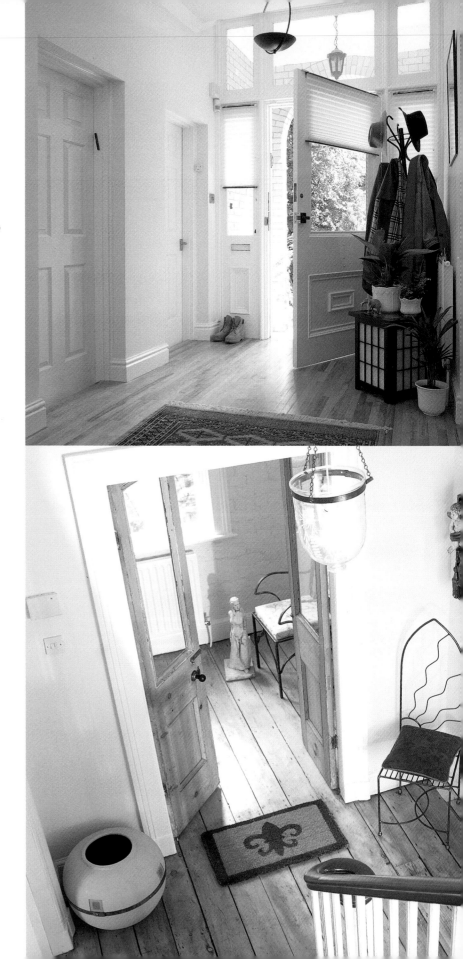

# **RUG***lore*

*R*ugs have long been artefacts of magic. It is said that dried seaweed, under a rug will improve finances; and that anyone who walks on an accidentally upturned rug will be blessed. The shape of a rug is believed to possess hidden influences.

✦ SQUARE OR RECTANGULAR RUGS—
THESE ARE BEST SUITED TO OFFICES,
LIBRARIES, DENS, AND THE HALLS
LEADING TO THESE ROOMS, AS THEY
REPRESENT THE MATERIAL WORLD,
INTELLECT, AND TECHNOLOGY.

✦ ROUND RUG—SYMBOLIZES
SPIRITUALITY AND PEACE, AND IS IN
SYMPATHY WITH THE QUIET
ENVIRONMENT OF A BEDROOM OR
RETREAT. A ROUND RUG MAY
ENCOURAGE A MORE PEACEFUL AND
CONVIVIAL ATMOSPHERE IN A LIVING
ROOM OR DINING ROOM.

✦ OVAL RUG—THE OVAL IS THE
SYMBOL OF THE COSMIC EGG, WHICH
IS THE ESSENCE OF ALL THAT EXISTS.
AN OVAL RUG CAN BE USED IN ANY
ROOM IN THE HOME.

✦ TO PURIFY AND SCENT A RUG, FIRST
SPRINKLE THE RUG WITH SALT AND
THEN TAKE IT OUTSIDE AND BEAT IT
WITH A BROOM. SCENT THE RUG BY
SCATTERING LAVENDER, ROSEMARY
OR OTHER SWEET-SMELLING HERBS
OVER IT. ROLL UP THE RUG TO
ALLOW THE SCENT TO PERMEATE,
AND THEN VACUUM OR SHAKE TO
REMOVE THE HERBS.

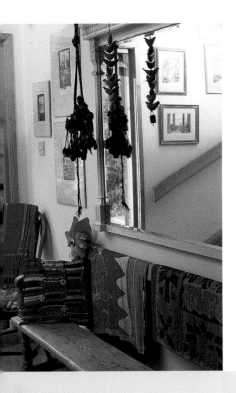

## DOORS, HALLWAYS, AND FENG SHUI

Ch'i energies enter a home through the front door, and the more often the threshold is crossed, the greater the flow of ch'i. This means that the entrance to a home is very influential. To insure that the ch'i energies entering your home are favorable, you must assess the location and aspect of the entrance, and choose door color and door furniture with care. You can, of course, correct unfavorable ch'i with trees and plants, winding paths, lighting, sculptures, and significant totems (see page 99).

When ch'i energy enters the home, it is the entrance hall that directs its movement and it is here that the first influence of its path can be applied. The ideal path for ch'i energy, once it enters the home, is to move smoothly and evenly into every room and then to exit from an opening somewhere near the front door.

*Two very different entrances (FAR LEFT AND LEFT) but both use feng shui tools— reflective surfaces, mirrors, chimes— to aid the progress of ch'i energy.*

> *"There's nothing worth the wear of winning,
> But laughter and the love of friends."*
>
> HILAIRE BELLOC

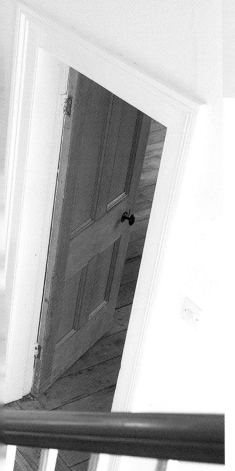

If an entrance hall is cluttered and poorly lit, the flow of ch'i will be blocked or will stagnate in the recesses caused by the clutter. A long and sparsely decorated hall will cause ch'i to stampede and have an unsettling effect on the ch'i in the rest of the home.

To decorate and design an entrance hall to encourage favorable ch'i, it may help to imagine ch'i as a body of moving air. The aim is to manipulate it so that it does not howl through the hall like a tornado that disturbs everything in its path, but rather moves like a zephyr that makes gentle, passing contact with everything but causes no turmoil.

To slow the flow of ch'i, use round-leafed, bushy plants, rugs, and subdued lighting. Mirrors will redirect ch'i so that it enters recesses and moves into other areas of the home. If you feel that ch'i is stagnating, excite it with lights, candles, wind chimes, or even a water feature.

*An L-shaped entrance (LEFT) that uses sculptures and natural light to stimulate ch'i.*

# *7 living* R O O M

Living rooms are often the least "alive" room of a home—full of synthetic carpets, polyurethane foam-filled sofas, and decorated with conventional paint or vinyl wallpaper. Creating a real "living" room means stripping out the synthetics and bringing in natural materials, which are health-giving and offer emotional warmth and spiritual uplift.

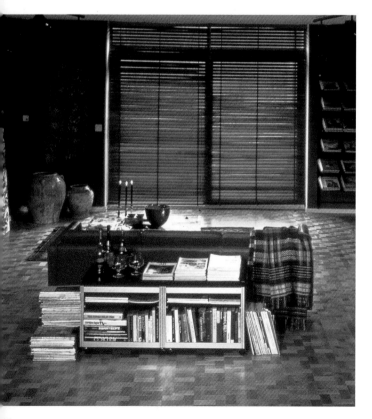

*Natural materials, a multitude of lighting options, and minimal furniture (ABOVE) create a functional and atmospheric living room.*

Wood floors scattered with rugs, and a minimum of furniture offer an uncluttered backdrop for all the activities we associate with living rooms—relaxing, entertaining, talking, reading, and playing. There should be sofas for sitting or reclining on that are arranged to encourage conversation and interaction rather than television-watching, a quiet corner for reading, and enough open floor area for children—and even adults!—to play in.

The best living rooms have plenty of natural light, with furniture or "play" areas positioned to take full advantage of it. You may also want to consider a layout that affords a good outlook into a garden or beyond. Young children, and anyone who is confined to the home, benefit greatly if they can, in even a passive way, interact with the wider world be it a garden or a busy street. It is of little wonder then that conservatories have become very popular in countries where winters can be long and summers short.

Artificial lighting should be flexible, but planned. Try out low-level lamps—table lamps and floor lamps—and uplights to create the atmosphere you want. You can even use lighting to create "rooms" within the living room—intimate lighting to define a conversation area, overhead lighting for a play area, and spotlights or downlights to draw attention to special features. A reading or meditation corner can also be delineated by the type of lighting used.

In the evening, candlelight will alter the mood, even when used in conjunction with artificial lighting. Match the color of the candle to your desired mood: orange candles to foster happiness and friendships, yellow to stimulate conversation, and blue and purple for peaceful mellowing and harmony.

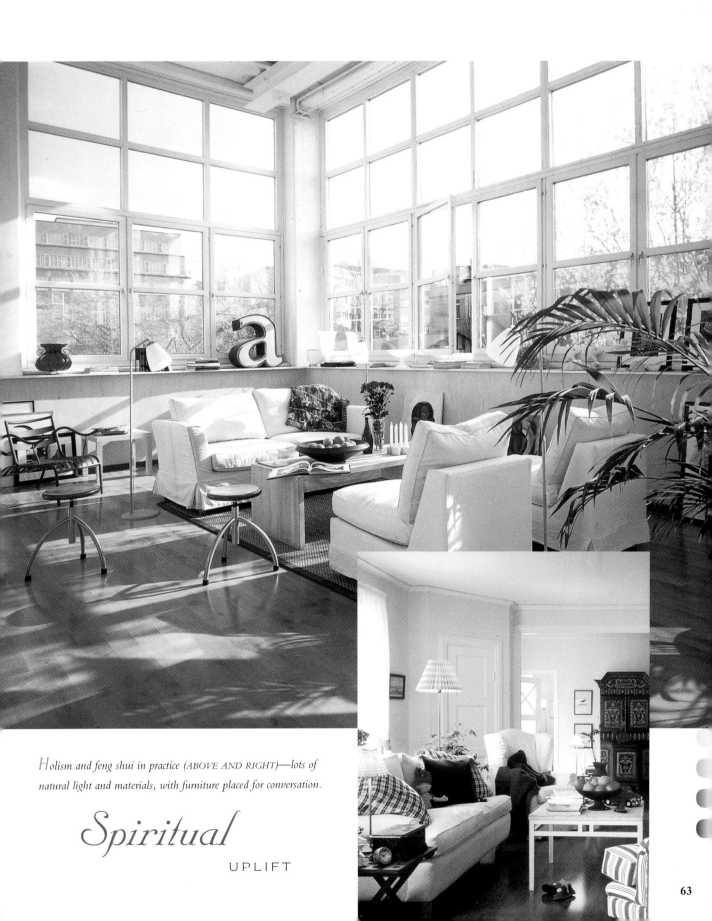

*Holism and feng shui in practice (ABOVE AND RIGHT)—lots of natural light and materials, with furniture placed for conversation.*

## Spiritual

### UPLIFT

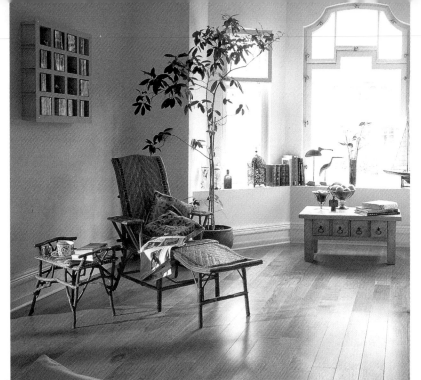

*W*e all benefit from taking the weight off
our feet once in a while (LEFT).

*H*olistic perfection (BELOW)—not a
synthetic surface or fabric in sight! A living
room that lives in every respect.

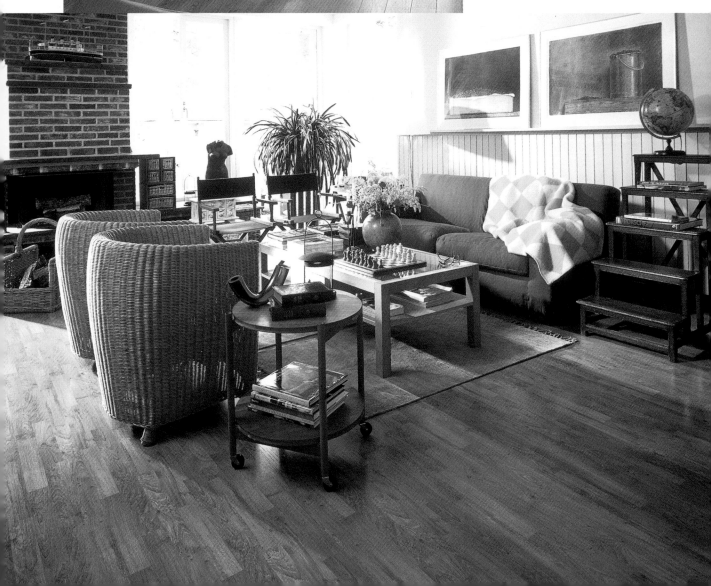

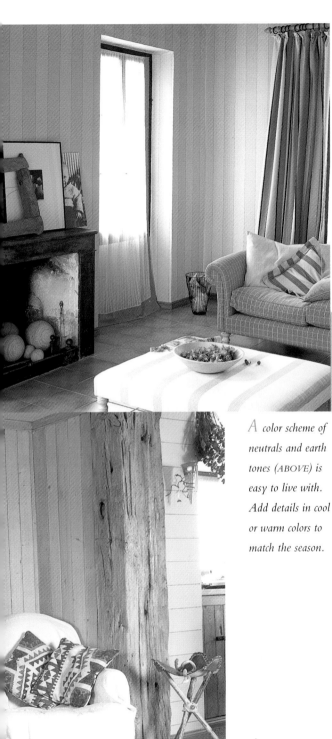

### Choosing furniture for comfort and posture

A good sofa or upholstered chair is made from natural materials, is comfortable, and is contoured to promote good posture. The key to good posture is ensuring the body is free of tension, and that there is support for the lumbar region of the spine. The seat, or base, needs to be firm to deter a slumped, round-shouldered posture, wide enough to support the back of the thighs, without digging into the back of the knees, and high enough to allow the feet to rest easily on the floor. A sofa with padded or wooden arms will help take the weight and stress of the neck, and provide support for people who have difficulties sitting or getting up from a seated position.

*Creating a real living room means stripping out the synthetics and bringing in the natural.*

*A color scheme of neutrals and earth tones (ABOVE) is easy to live with. Add details in cool or warm colors to match the season.*

We relax best when there is an angle of more than 90 degrees between the hips and the lumbar region of the spine. The back of the sofa should support the whole spine as well as the neck and head. Rocking chairs and porch-swing loungers are particularly good in these respects.

Reclining, rather than sitting, is more comfortable if you suffer from back problems. And everyone benefits from a padded footstool or ottoman that allows you literally to take the weight off your feet. Specific leg aches may be eased if the feet are higher than the hips. A chair with a tilting mechanism and adjustable settings is perfect for older people and anyone with a physical disability.

The final pre-requisite for a comfortable sofa or chair is a natural fabric covering. Natural fabrics breathe, making them more accommodating in hot weather especially.

*A favorite chair (LEFT) has been stripped of synthetic fabrics and draped in a cotton throw.*

*Emotional*
WARMTH

65

*A tranquil and contemplative corner of a south-west facing living room (RIGHT).*

## FENG SHUI IN THE LIVING ROOM

The critical elements of living room feng shui are space, position, and layout. Ch'i will stagnate in an overcrowded room, and if that means knocking two rooms together to make one generous room, it will be worth it. If such a solution is not possible, then employ the tools mentioned on pages 68-69 to unblock ch'i.

Where you sit can affect your relationships with others, your attitude and your well-being. There are two factors to take into account: the direction you face, and the position of your sofa or chair. How the seating is grouped will also influence atmosphere. Of these, though, direction is the most influential. Use the specific ch'i energies related to each direction to solve problems or to help you achieve something. A chair, positioned in the north-west is auspicious for motivation, yet if the chair is facing south-west a cautious attitude will prevail. These seemingly conflicting energies result in a pragmatic energy.

*The critical elements of living room feng shui are space, position, and layout.*

Seating should be grouped around a low table to form a square, rectangle or circle. Any side not occupied with a sofa or chair can be filled with a plant, a special feature, or a side table. Enclosing the seating in this way will promote harmony. If you work in positions where communication skills are paramount then arrange yourself to be sitting in the south-east facing north-west. If romance is what you seek, take a seat facing west. The longer you spend in a particular seating location, the greater the influence.

## *Sociable*

AMBIENCE

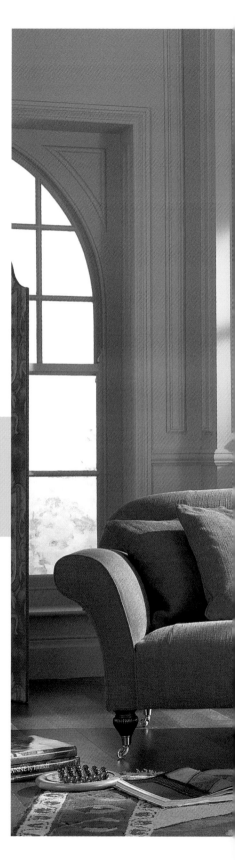

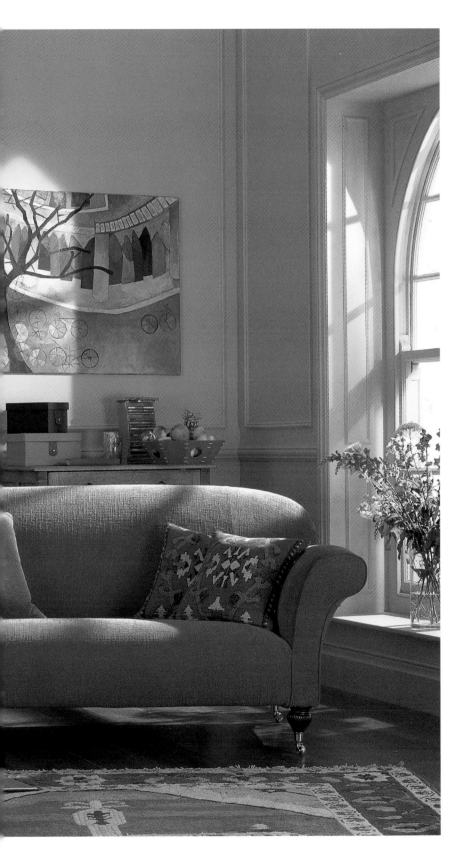

# SUNLIGHT *in your life*

*S*unlight *contributes to creating a lively, happy living space, so the position of your living room in relation to the movement of the Sun is important. Most favorable positions are those that are south, south-east, south-west, and west of the physical center of your home.*

✦ South—this aspect has a warm, sociable atmosphere that may call for calming touches. Balance the energetic ch'i with soft shades of purple and touches of pale yellow. Geometric prints on fabrics, rugs, wall finishes, or evident other decoration will enhance ch'i.

✦ South-east—lively ch'i energy is complemented by shades of green and blue, and because the living room is beautifully light, you can consider using dark green. Vertical stripes or irregular patterns will support ch'i.

✦ South-west—offers a settled and domestic atmosphere, which is enhanced with earth colors like yellow or brown to create a cosy and relaxed ambience. Splashes of purple will add to ch'i, as will checkered or angular patterns.

✦ West—a naturally joyous and pleasurable location. Curved patterns on fabric, rugs or wall finishes in soft reds and pinks with touches of grey and white will support the natural energies.

# LIVING *atmosphere*

*Experiment with essential oil-scented spray mists and candles, or essential oil burners to create exactly the right atmosphere in your living room. Use orange, mandarin and pine to uplift and refresh; bergamot to calm; and juniper to purify and stimulate.*

✦ TO MAINTAIN HARMONIOUS CH'I, SPIKY PLANTS LIKE YUCCAS SHOULD BE AVOIDED IN LIVING ROOMS—AND, IN FACT, IN ANY ROOM IN THE HOME—UNLESS THEY ARE SURROUNDED BY PLENTY OF SPACE. SPIKY PLANTS, LIKE SHARP EDGES, CUT CH'I.

✦ A COSY, OPEN FIRE IS A NATURAL FOCAL POINT IN LIVING ROOM, AND HAS FOR ALMOST EVERY CULTURE ALWAYS SYMBOLIZED THE HEART OF THE HOME. IT MAY BE A WASTEFUL, POLLUTING, AND INEFFICIENT WAY OF HEATING A ROOM, BUT THE PLEASURE OF WATCHING THE FLAMES LEAP AND FLICKER, RELAXING IN THE COMFORT THEY OFFER, AND THE LINK IT GIVES TO OUR ANCESTORS, MAKE OPEN FIRES HIGHLY DESIRABLE.

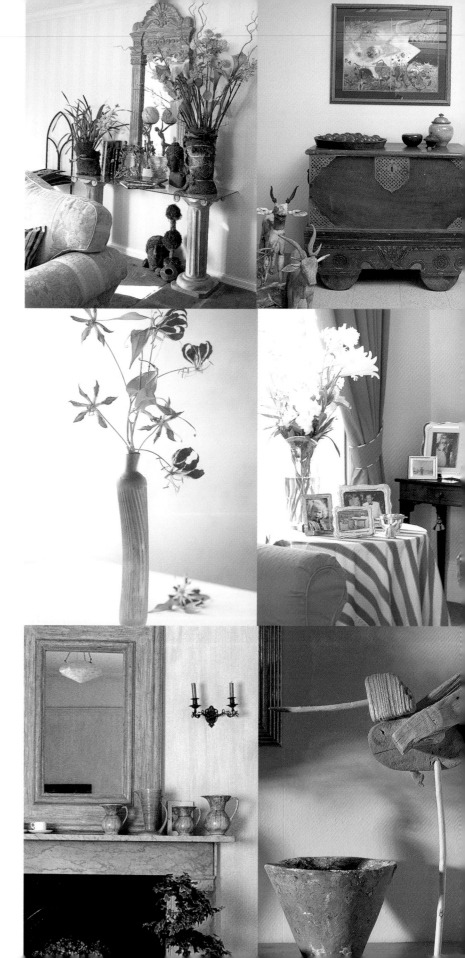

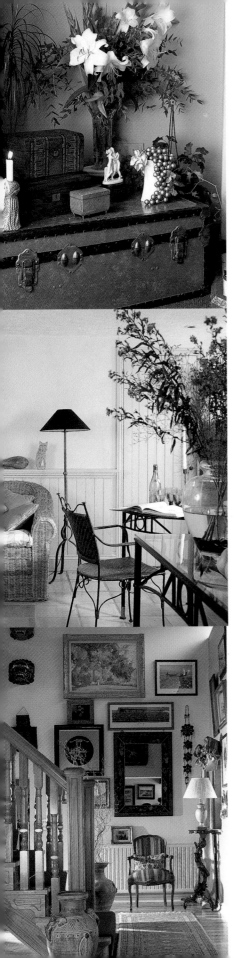

### Decorating details for ch'i

Every element in a room will have a bearing on the flow of ch'i. Ch'i can be influenced by color, pattern, shape, position, and the material from which the object is made. Following are some tools you can use to manipulate ch'i—to correct bad energy, to stimulate ch'i, or simply to enhance it. But the object alone is not sufficient, you must employ it in the right place to have the desired effect.

✦ Square boxes of wood and metal—add metal energy and should be used in a south-west position to boost stability.

✦ Metal picture frames—hung or standing in the north-west or west of the living room will add solid metal energy.

✦ Clay objects—to foster a steady atmosphere, place them in the north-east.. To foster family harmony, use squat clay or plaster statues in black, white or yellow.

✦ Glazed ceramics—if spherical or rounded they will help concentrate ch'i energy in the north and east.

✦ Clear glass objects like vases and bottles—encourage smooth flow of ch'i in the north—an aspect usually lacking in direct natural light— of a room.

✦ Wooden sculptures of animals—to add liveliness, particularly effective in east and south-east positions.

✦ Irregularly-shaped glass objects—place in the north of a room for peace and tranquility.

✦ Metal statues with a romantic theme—position in the west of the room, or even the garden, to kindle love.

*Decorating details for manipulating and fostering specific ch'i energies (LEFT TO RIGHT FROM TOP): romantic metal sculpture, metal frame, and sculptures in clay; hand-carved wooden deer; trinket boxes and chest made from wood and metal; organic-shaped glass vase; silver picture frames; cat sculpture and clear glass vase; glazed ceramics over the fireplace; clay and wood animal sculpture and pot; large clay pots.*

# 8 kitchen

The kitchen is the holistic heart of the home. The best are more than simply places where we cook and eat: they are the warm and inviting social hub of the home. An holistic kitchen is one you don't want to leave!

In creating a holistic kitchen, you need to look not only at its function—food preparation, storage, and consumption—but also at the ways you can reduce waste and pollution, and give this hard-working room a positive atmosphere.

*Maximize storage with flexible solutions like string bags, or build shelves in an empty corner (BELOW). String bags are perfect for storing vegetables and fruit—the fibers breathe and air can circulate preventing dampness and early rotting.*

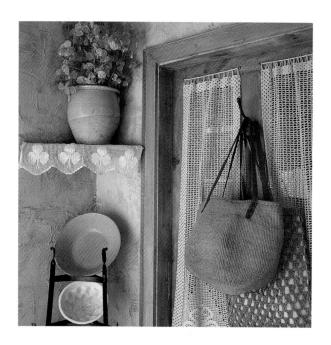

In practical terms, an holistic kitchen needs to have plentiful and appropriate storage space for home-grown produce and for the short-term storage of newspapers, aluminum cans, and other materials destined for re-use or recycling. Organic matter for the compost pile needs to kept in a washable, lidded container. To empty cupboards, suspend pots and pans from butcher's hooks, and cups and mugs from wooden pegs. Terracotta plant pots are great for storing cutlery, as well as providing easy access. Cotton or net string bags can be used to store produce, and plastic bags, cloth, and paper that will be re-used. The bags can be hung on the inside of cupboards, on the back of a door or, if so fortunate, in a pantry, larder, or large store cupboard that is vented to the outside.

A kitchen that "works" is also kind to those who work in it. Work surfaces need to be at a height that allows you to maintain a good posture whatever you are doing: higher work surfaces for chopping, lower for kneading. In existing kitchens, tricks such as a solid wooden step to reduce the height and a thick chopping board to increase the height of a work surface can be employed.

Make good use of any natural light, and restrict harsh lighting to food preparation areas. Downlights over preparation areas are perfect. Experiment with softer lighting and candles in an eating area or quiet corner.

A kitchen should also be ergonomic. This means that the stove and oven, refrigerator, and sink are positioned for easy access and each within easy reach of the other. A kitchen that demands a half-marathon sprint between stove and sink, for example, is not doing you any favors.

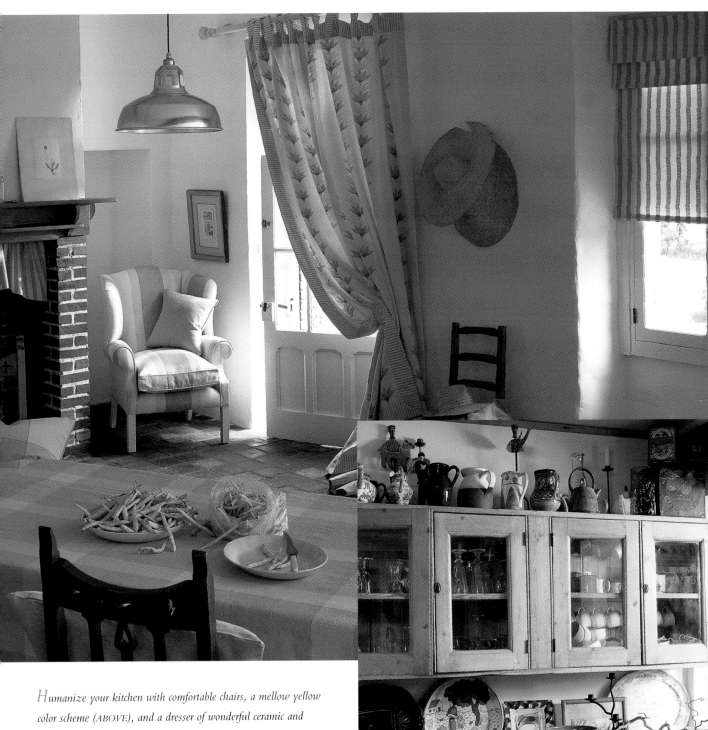

*H*umanize your kitchen with comfortable chairs, a mellow yellow color scheme (ABOVE), and a dresser of wonderful ceramic and stoneware dishes (RIGHT).

*Inviting*

WARM

# THE SAFE
## *kitchen*

*W*hile most of us would like to consider that the kitchen should be the most hygienic and holistic room, it is often also the repository for many hazardous products and things on their way to a recycling facility. Following are useful facts about recycling.

◆ NEVER DISPOSE OF ANY OF THE FOLLOWING PRODUCTS IN HOUSEHOLD GARBAGE—AMMONIA-BASED CLEANERS, BLEACH, PETROCHEMICAL-BASED CLEANSERS, DRAIN CLEANSERS, OVEN CLEANERS, FLOOR POLISH, CARPET CLEANERS, MEDICINES, ACETONE (NAIL POLISH REMOVER), BATTERIES, SYNTHETIC OR OIL-BASE PAINTS, GARDEN PESTICIDES OR FUNGICIDES, WEED KILLERS, AEROSOL CANS, MOTOR OIL, EPOXY ADHESIVES, PAINT THINNERS OR WHITE SPIRIT. CONTACT YOUR LOCAL AUTHORITIES FOR DETAILS OF WHERE TO DISPOSE OF THESE HAZARDOUS MATERIALS.

◆ THESE CAN ALL BE RECYCLED AT LOCAL FACILITIES—ALUMINUM CANS AND FOIL PRODUCTS, METALS, NATURAL FIBERS AND FABRICS, AND PAPER AND CARDBOARD PRODUCTS.

◆ CONTACT LOCAL AUTHORITIES FOR SPECIFIC RECYCLING LOCATIONS— TIRES, BUILDING MATERIALS, CAR BATTERIES, OLD ENGINE OIL, AND PAINT.

◆ MANY PLASTICS WILL NOT BIODEGRADE NO MATTER WHAT IS DONE WITH THEM. AVOID BUYING SUCH PLASTICS ENTIRELY. PLASTICS THAT CAN BE RECYCLED WILL BE CLEARLY LABELED.

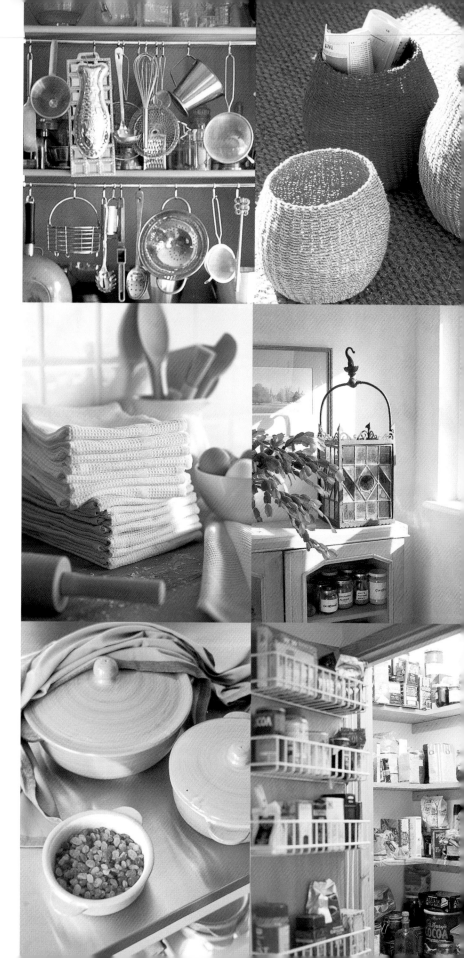

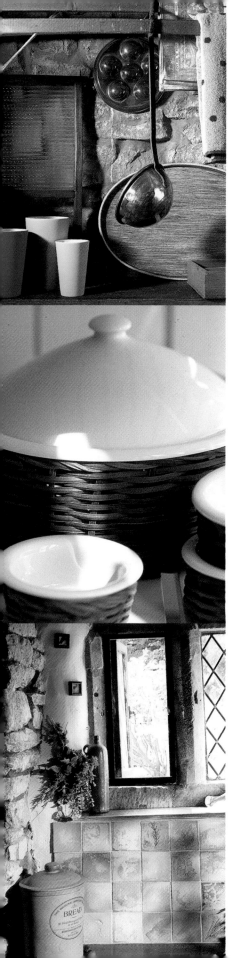

## How green is your kitchen?

The essence of a "green" kitchen is one that is energy-efficient and health-promoting. Replace old and inefficient white goods and appliances with those given a high energy-efficiency rating, or substitute standard electrical plugs with those that restrict the amount of electricity supplied to the amount actually required by the appliance. This simple and inexpensive modification can reduce energy-consumption by up to 20 percent. But the greatest energy-saving change is to reduce your reliance on kitchen gadgets. Water is precious, so fix low-flow taps to reduce water consumption.

Energy-efficiency also means recycling. Buy only what you need, and when making a purchase consider whether it can be re-used or recycled when its original purpose is finished. Glass, aluminum cans, and all paper products (including cellophane) can be recycled over and over again by environmentally friendly and energy-efficient processes. Paper products are also naturally biodegradable. Tin-plated steel cans can be recycled, but the resulting metal is of a poor quality, and facilities for recycling plastic are, at present, inadequate. Organic matter—vegetable peelings, uncooked food, and egg-shells—make good compost for your plants.

A health-promoting kitchen is devoid of materials that give off toxic fumes, or that will react with other substances to produce dangerous by-products. Aluminum can leach into foods cooked in aluminum pots or pans, and unlined copper pans—-if not thoroughly cleaned—will accumulate toxic verdigris. Some non-stick coatings can also contaminate food and are best avoided. Good alternatives are stainless steel, toughened glass, cast iron, enamel, and oven-proof earthenware. Earthenware and unpainted stoneware are best for table and serving flatware, and smooth stainless steel for cutlery.

*An holistic kitchen is not just healthy and holistic, it is brimming with things that are lovely to work with, handle, and behold (LEFT).*

A water filter will remove nitrates, lead, and organic substances such as pesticides from tap water. Under-sink filters are efficient, and water filter jugs are inexpensive. But whichever one you choose to use, the filter cartridges must be changed frequently. A choked filter will introduce more nasties into the water than there were originally. Store filter jugs in the refrigerator and wash them weekly to prevent bacterial contamination. Water for babies' feeds should always be boiled.

Filters in stove hoods or extractor fans should also be changed or cleaned regularly.

Dispose of hazardous waste, for example bleach or scouring powder, carefully. Products like these will contaminate the water supply. Better still, use only natural, non-toxic cleaning products that are totally biodegradable.

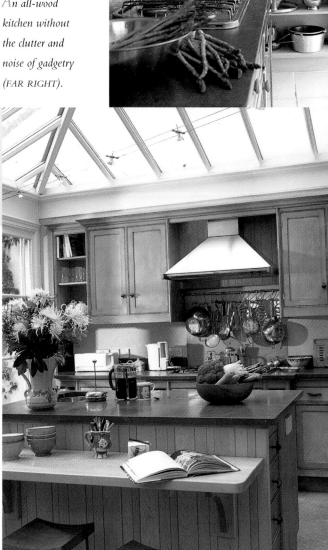

*Stainless steel equipment and surfaces are very hygienic (RIGHT) and ch'i is activated by its reflective finish.*

*An all-wood kitchen without the clutter and noise of gadgetry (FAR RIGHT).*

## Food preparation is believed to be influenced by the surrounding ch'i energy

### FENG SHUI IN THE KITCHEN

Eating healthily is an important part of traditional Chinese medicine, and food preparation is believed to be influenced by the surrounding ch'i energy. A kitchen therefore needs to be sited east or south-east of the center of the home so that the two incompatible elements of fire (the stove and oven) and water (the sink and automatic dishwasher) are harmonized. Ideally, fire and water elements should not be next to each other, but separated by earth elements like plants, and earthenware or stoneware containers.

Blues or greens are favored colors, with dashes of yellow and purple. Add patterns based on leaves, vegetables, and fruit in blinds and other fabrics, and decorative features.

Ch'i is activated by shiny surfaces like tiles and stainless steel, and spotlights directed into awkward corners will prevent stagnating ch'i. Wooden flooring and furniture are recommended in the kitchen.

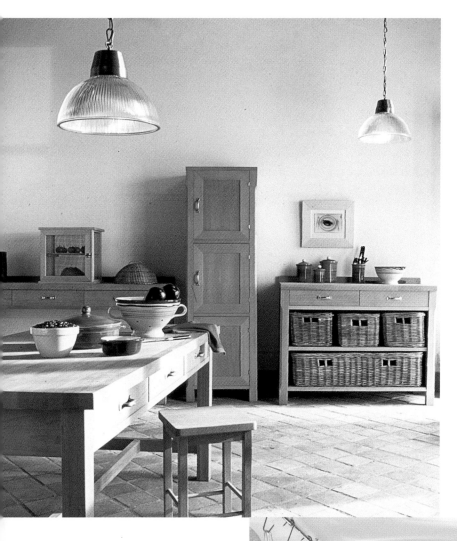

*L*emons set to absorb cooking odours, while
a vase of flowers helps clean and humidify
the air (BELOW).

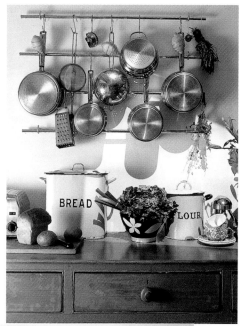

*B*lue with accents of yellow is a favored
color scheme for a feng shui kitchen (LEFT).
The energies here will also benefit from
abundant natural light.

*A* clay sculpture introduces a vital earth
element to separate water and fire elements,
and downlights will prevent ch'i stagnating
under the cupboards (RIGHT).

# THE CHARMED
## *kitchen*

*In every aspect the kitchen should tantalize and therefore charm the senses. You should have the pleasure of working with tools that are pleasing to touch, and on surfaces that are natural. You should be surrounded by colors, smells, and light that negate the downside of kitchen chores.*

*The spider plant (RIGHT) helps control humidity and clean the air, but its hanging fronds conceal a sharp corner that would cut ch'i.*

*A rope of garlic (LEFT) or chiles is believed to absorb evil spirits.*

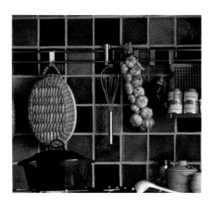

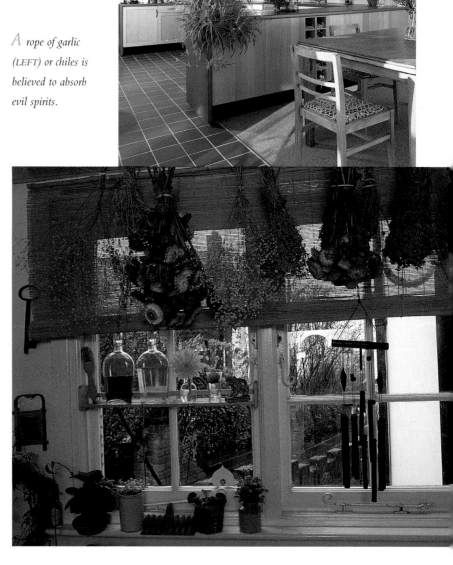

- ✦ YELLOW IS A WONDERFUL KITCHEN COLOR THAT ENCOURAGES PEOPLE TO GATHER ROUND. INTRODUCE YEAR-ROUND SCENT AND TEXTURE BY GROWING HERBS, PLANTS, OR PRODUCE ON A WINDOW LEDGE. THE ALOE PLANT IS SAID TO PROTECT THE COOK, AND ITS MATURE LEAVES PRODUCE A GEL THAT RELIEVES A PAINFUL BURN.

- ✦ CREATE A CORNER FOR YOURSELF IN THE KITCHEN AND MARK OUT THIS NO-WORK TERRITORY WITH FRESH FLOWERS, A CANDLE OR ESSENTIAL OIL BURNER (LEMON ESSENTIAL OIL WILL REFRESH AND UPLIFT), AND A TREASURED OBJECT. RETREAT INTO YOUR SPECIAL AREA TO INVIGORATE OR RELAX.

*A charmed kitchen (ABOVE) with herbs and flowers, homemade oils, and wind chime.*

# 9 dining ROOM

We must eat to live, so the act of eating is vested with great significance; and sharing a meal with others is said to create unique bonds. Indeed, ritual meals form the basis of many religions and cultural celebrations. A room where we eat, then, is a setting for something of great importance, and should be decorated with care.

It does not matter if you have a separate dining room, or if your kitchen or living room doubles as a dining area. Feng shui recommends that it is important to set aside a particular area for dining to ensure that the household gather together in what should be a harmonizing event. If a separate dining room is unused for a period, scent it with lemon, grapefruit, mandarin or orange essential oils to keep the atmosphere fresh and inviting.

A meal is a very sensual experience that can excite all the senses. So it is not only important to whet the appetite with glorious food that smells as good as it tastes, but to set a table that looks and feels wonderful. There is, in this respect, little to compare with wooden dining furniture that is not hidden under a cloth, nor smothered with distracting elements.

Some believe that a dining room table should stand parallel to the walls so that the lines of energy, believed to run through the home's foundations, will flow smoothly around the table. Others contend that a round table is better because it is inclusive and affords no-one "head of the table" status.

Red in a dining room will stimulate appetite, say the color therapists. Alternatively, yellow or orange are very sociable colors that work well in any room where people gather. Orange candles on the table will encourage enthusiasm and a feeling of togetherness.

*This simply laid, bare wooden table (BELOW) in a light-filled room shows that "decorating with care" does not mean gilding the lily.*

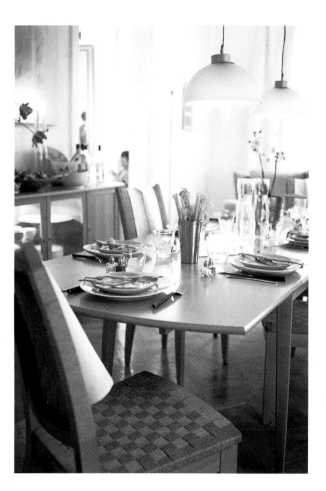

## Sociable

TOGETHERNESS

## THE LORE *of wood*

Different types of wood are believed to be imbued with magical influences. It is a pity that this magic has not affected the forests from which the timbers are gleaned. Hardwood timber forests, for example, are denuded and replanted with fast-growing pines. A star alongside any of the following indicates that a timber is currently regarded as under threat.

✦ CEDAR—HEALING, LONGEVITY, PROTECTION, AND PURIFICATION

✦ CHERRY—LOVE

✦ EBONY—MAGICAL POWER AND PROTECTION

✦ MAHOGANY—PROTECTION AGAINST LIGHTNING

✦ MAPLE—LOVE AND, MONEY

✦ OAK—HEALTH, LUCK, PROTECTION, AND STRENGTH

✦ PINE—EXORCISM, HEALING, AND MONEY

✦ RATTAN★—LUCK AND STRENGTH

✦ REDWOOD—LONGEVITY

✦ TEAK★—RICHES

✦ WALNUT—HEALTH

*Fresh lemons (RIGHT) or lemon essential oil are the perfect scent for a dining area.*

*A separate dining room is not necessary. It is far more important that a dining area is inviting and encourages interaction (BELOW).*

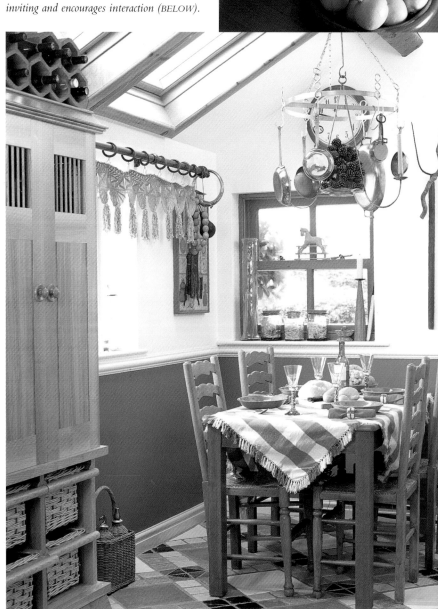

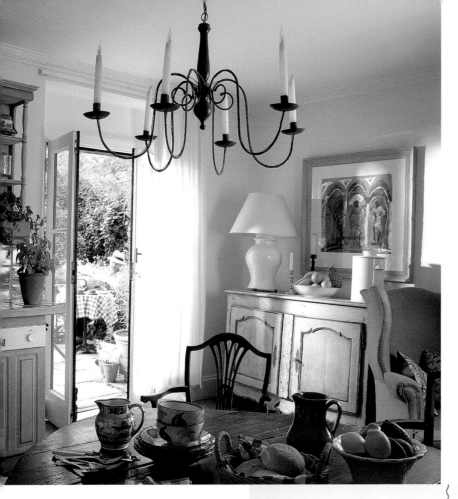

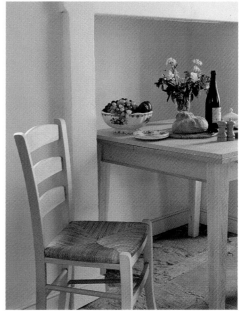

*A straight-back wooden chair (ABOVE)
promotes a good eating posture.*

*A round table (ABOVE) is a great leveler—
no-one can dominate or crown themselves
"head of the table".*

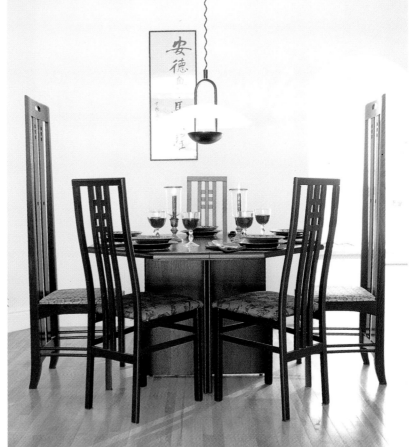

*A formal dining room (RIGHT) where
decoration is minimal so as to concentrate
energies on the ritual of sharing a meal. A
low, overhead light further focuses attention.*

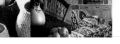

## FENG SHUI AT THE TABLE

Particularly good locations for a dining area are east, south-east and north-west of the center of the home. Depending on your lifestyle, you may prefer to breakfast by the morning Sun, or dine by a setting Sun when ch'i energy blesses entertaining, romance, and pleasure. Use greens and blues in easterly and south-easterly dining rooms; pinks and reds in a west location; and grays or white in the north-west.

A round dining table is harmonious and encourages relaxation, with wood the preferred material. Feng shui graces pine with informal qualities, and mahogany for formal situations. A square or rectangular table can be angled so that people sit where they feel more comfortable and linked to their ch'i energy.

Shiny platters, candle holders, sparkling glasses, and cutlery will stimulate ch'i making for a more enlivening yang atmosphere. Unglazed earthen flatware will slow ch'i. As a rule of thumb—formal (or more yang) settings are minimal and uncluttered and typified by hard, shiny surfaces.

Certain colors are also associated with mood and energies. Use cream table settings for a relaxing meal, blue or green to stimulate communication, pink or red for romance and passion, and yellow to evoke warm, familial feelings. As very few of us possess more than the necessary flatware, create the mood you want by varying the color of napkins, candles, table mats, flowers, or a display of fruit and vegetables in the appropriate color.

*A dining setting with a gently curved table, and wonderful aspect. The mood could be dramatically altered and ch'i manipulated.*

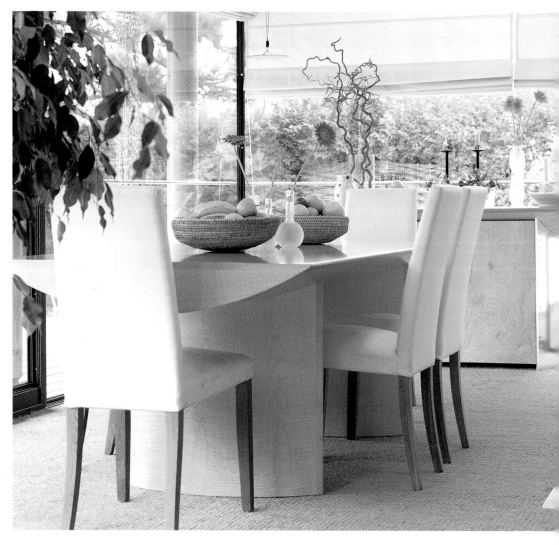

# 10 study, den,

## H O M E   O F F I C E

A home work-space should be designed to help you work efficiently in a healthy and invigorating environment. It should be a quiet room away from the hubbub of household activities, and one that can be closed off from the rest of home. This will provide necessary solitude, and allow the user literally to "shut the door" on work or study. Making this clear physical, emotional, and mental distinction between work and living areas is vital, especially now that so many people are opting to run their working lives from home.

If a separate study or den is not feasible, designate an area in the living room for this use. Never convert part of your bedroom, as it is difficult to create an atmosphere that is conducive to work and sleep.

### Combining function and comfort

The key items are a desk and chair. The height of the desk must be appropriate for the work you do, and the chair should support the small of the back. To meet the physical needs of all those who use it, a chair with adjustable height and backrest is best. Though it will be more expensive, the health benefits of maintaining good posture and avoiding backache are well worth it. If you are using a computer, make sure you are sitting so that your fingers and palms rest easily on the keyboard or mouse. Your elbows should be bent at right angles.

The desk—as large as possible—should be near a window so that natural light and ventilation are excellent, with window dressings tied back so as not to obstruct a single ray of light or whisper of wind. Artificial lighting, using daylight bulbs, should be flexible, throwing gentle light where needed but not causing glare on computer screens or eye strain.

*Paramount considerations when siting and planning a work environment are good lighting and ventilation (BELOW).*

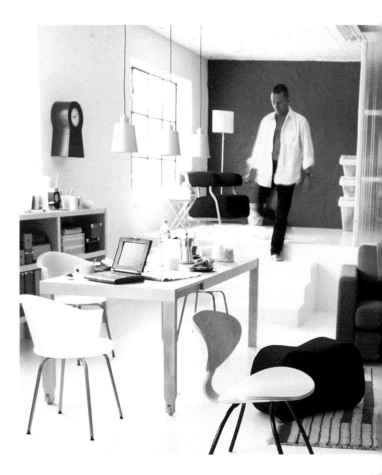

*Invigorating*

HEALTHY

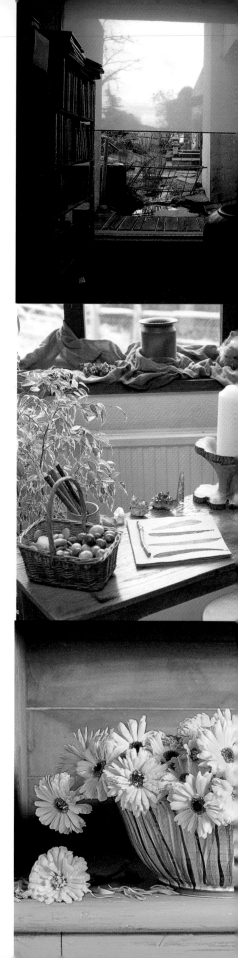

Careful consideration of these elements is the basis of a physically comfortable environment; a healthy environment means stripping out artificial materials and stripping back synthetic and petrochemical-based finishes. Reduce the electromagnetic field (EMF) around a computer with an EMF shield, and always sit as far away from the screen as you can, and avoid working to the left and right of the screen where the EMF is greatest.

Office electrical equipment that is switched on for long periods—some never turned off—dries the atmosphere and fills it with positive ions, and papers and books radically increase the dust and dustmite count. Counter by maintaining the humidity—and at the same time doing your attitude no end of good—with bowls of water, vases of flowers, and pots of scented plants. Storing papers and books behind closed doors, a drape or blind, will reduce dust and keep distracting clutter out of sight. Feng shui also advises against open shelves as their recesses cause ch'i to stagnate.

### Attention to detail

To be efficient and inspired in your work or study, pay attention to the small things. Is there something wonderful to look at when you raise your eyes from a book or from the computer screen? Is the furniture and decoration so functional that it saps, rather than stimulates? Is there a corner in the study where you can take a step back from your work in order to get a new perspective on it?

It is possible to introduce emotion into this room without sacrificing practicalities. Yellow, according to color therapists, stimulates the intellect and encourages communication, so even if a room make-over is out of the question, add splashes of yellow in flowering plants, a rug, a throw over the chair, or even by swapping white stationery for yellow. And to relieve the visual tedium of bland and uniformly colored office equipment, use patterned and textured fabrics.

A study is the perfect place for an aquarium. The water will help humidify the air, and research has confirmed that watching the slow and graceful movements of fish, is calming and will reduce blood pressure. As talismans, fish are said to bring love and blessings; goldfish are believed to attract money, and repulse negative energies.

*Surround yourself with beautiful natural objects, textures, sights, and scents, and air purifying plants (RIGHT). Very simple changes will make all the difference to your work environment.*

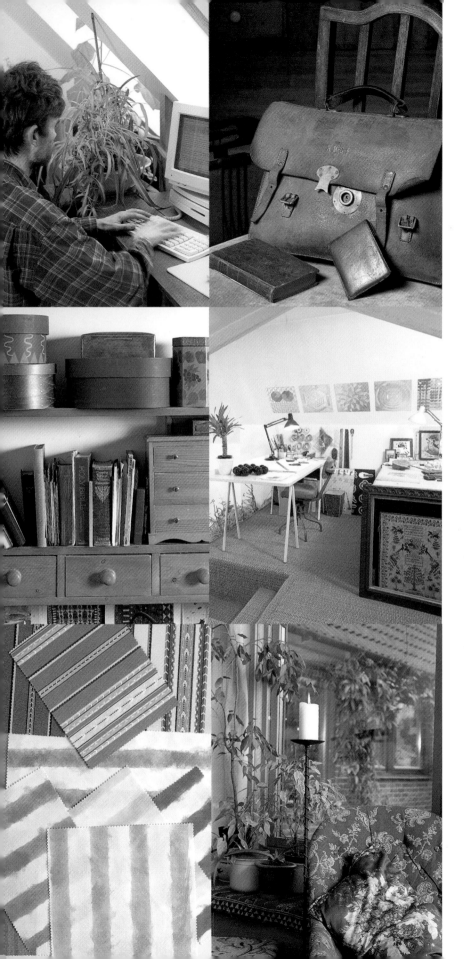

## ENERGIES *for work*

◆ PEPPERMINT, ROSEMARY, BASIL, AND
BERGAMOT ESSENTIAL OILS WILL AID
CONCENTRATION. USE AS A SPRAY
MIST DILUTED IN PURIFIED WATER,
OR BURN IN AN OIL BURNER.

◆ FOR CLARITY OF THOUGHT, PLACE
WIND CHIMES INSIDE THE DOOR OF
THE STUDY OR DEN, AND KEEP THE
ENTRANCE CLEAR. DO NOT USE THE
AREA BEHIND THE DOOR FOR
STORAGE—THE DOOR SHOULD BE
ABLE TO OPEN TO ITS FULL EXTENT,
LEST YOU HINDER THE ACCESS OF
OPPORTUNITY AND PROGRESS.

◆ CLEAN AND CLEAR THE DESK OF
UNNECESSARY CLUTTER AND DEBRIS
BEFORE COMMENCING ANY CREATIVE
TASK AND WHEN YOU HAVE FINISHED
WORKING FOR THE DAY.

◆ A VASE OF FLOWERS ON YOUR DESK
AND A ROUND MIRROR ON THE
WALL WILL BRING GOOD LUCK AND
LOVE INTO THE ROOM.

◆ CLEAN DOOR FURNITURE AND OIL
AWAY SQUEAKS, TO MAKE THE WAY
CLEAR FOR NEW OPPORTUNITIES.

83

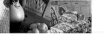

## FENG SHUI GOES TO WORK

The best locations for a study are east, south-east, south, and north-west of the center of the home. East is particularly good for new businesses and for putting ideas into practice; south-east has a similar ch'i energy, but it is calmer and better suited for consolidation and growth. A room in the south quarter will help attract attention and acclaim and in the north-west will inspire respect, leadership qualities, and organization.

To further manipulate ch'i, use blues and greens to decorate an east or south-east study; purple in a south location; and white and grays, with a dash of yellow in a north-west situation. Vertical stripes in fabric, paint effects or wallpaper will support ch'i.

What your desk is made from, and its size and shape, affect ch'i energy. The most auspicious energies are associated with a large, round or rounded desk made of wood. A rounded shape will not cut across or interrupt the flow of ch'i.

The layout of a study or office, and even of the desk itself, should conform to the nine trigrams of the ba-gua. For example, in the study you should emphasize wealth, fame, career, and knowledge positions. This can be done with crystals, heavy objects, wind chimes, or with objects linked to particular energies.

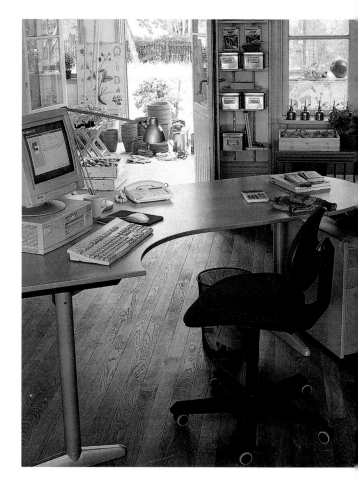

𝒩

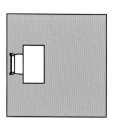

**FACING EAST**—FAVORS QUICK STARTS AND FAST GROWTH. IDEAL FOR ANYONE STARTING A NEW CAREER OR BUSINESS.

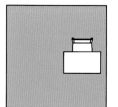

**FACING SOUTH**—SUPPORTIVE OF THOSE WORKING IN PROMOTIONS OR SALES, BUT NOT GOOD IF YOU ARE PRONE TO RESTLESSNESS.

𝒲 ———————————————————————————— 𝓔

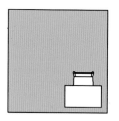

**FACING SOUTH WEST**—A CLASSIC POSITION FOR A TOP MANAGER. THE ENERGY INFLUENCES WILL ENHANCE LEADERSHIP AND DIGNITY.

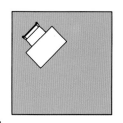

**SITTING SOUTH-EAST AND FACING SOUTH**—ACTIVATES GOOD COMMUNICATION AND IS SUITED TO LAWYERS, BUT INADVISABLE FOR ANYONE WHO IS EASILY EXCITED.

𝒮

# *bedroom*

A bedroom is a place of retreat, a welcoming and comforting sanctuary at any time of the day, not just at night. It should be a totally healthy environment and reflect the needs of its inhabitants more than any other room in the home.

Fufilling these needs is even more important if the bedroom is for an older, disabled or infirm person who may spend much more time in bed than any other member of the household—except, perhaps a teenager who in their prime seems to be either in bed asleep or holding court with their friends from their duvet-draped throne.

So what are the priorities—functional, health-imbued or spiritual—when decorating and designing a bedroom? Top of the list should be good ventilation and a toxin-free environment, maximizing natural light, and a good bed and bedding that assure comfortable sleep without causing backache or an allergic reaction.

Next comes creating a tranquil atmosphere by using feng shui and holistically inspired natural furnishings and decoration, sympathetic artificial lighting, and scent. Even teenagers should be encouraged to see their bedroom as somewhere to wind down, not just wind up the music.

That last point brings up the need to locate and to make bedrooms as quiet as possible. Furnishings, rugs, and the careful placement of bookshelves and wardrobes can help to dampen noise within the room and also defend it against external noise. To further decrease the intrusion of outside noises, hang thick, heavy drapes for night-time use and install double-glazing on windows.

There is one other option—relocate the room. Ignore all the current precepts about the designated functions of particular rooms, and let in some lateral thinking. If you have a den or spare room that is quiet, well ventilated and filled with natural light, transform it into a bedroom.

*Devoid of electrical appliances and synthetic fibers, this blue and lilac bedroom is warmed by soft natural light giving it a meditative atmosphere. By night, the crystals will catch flickering candlelight.*

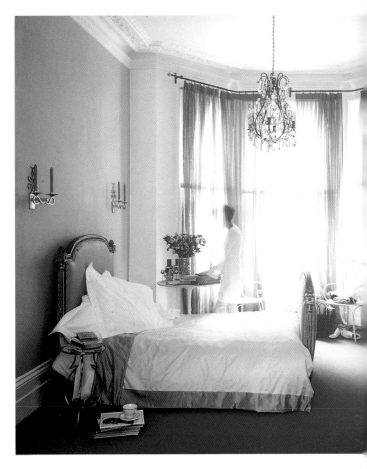

### Bedroom basics

Ideally a bedroom should be large enough to move about in easily, though the reality is often very different; from brownstone tenement block to modern detached, the cry is always the same—the bedrooms are too small!

But have you looked critically at how much valuable floor space is taken up with unnecessary furniture—for example, two bedside tables when only one is needed, freestanding chests of drawers rashly purchased to absorb the overflow from a wardrobe, a table upon which to stand a television—this list can go on and on. So before thinking evil thoughts about your home's original architect, do a spring clean and tackle the clutter. You should pay special attention to furniture made with particle board or composition board or painted with conventional synthetic paints. These items are filling the air with formaldehyde and other unwanted fumes.

A sense of space in even the smallest room can be created by replacing synthetic carpet with pale-colored, unstained wood flooring, and by using light-colored paints, fabrics, and bedding. The greatest space-maker is to use natural light to the fullest possible extent. This airy feeling can be replicated at night by artificial light that fills recesses and reflects off light-colored surfaces. Avoid dark furniture or features—they will absorb light.

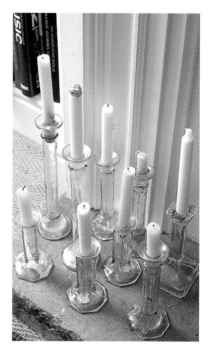

*Candles are wonderful in the bedroom at the end of the day (LEFT), but remember to extinguish them!*

*Romantic though it may be to slumber in a four-poster (RIGHT), a good mattress and bedding made of natural materials is critical.*

# *Tranquil*
SANCTUARY

*Wood flooring (RIGHT) is both a health option and one that makes a room seem light and spacious.*

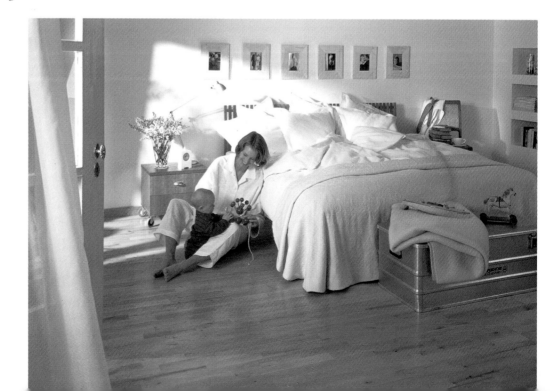

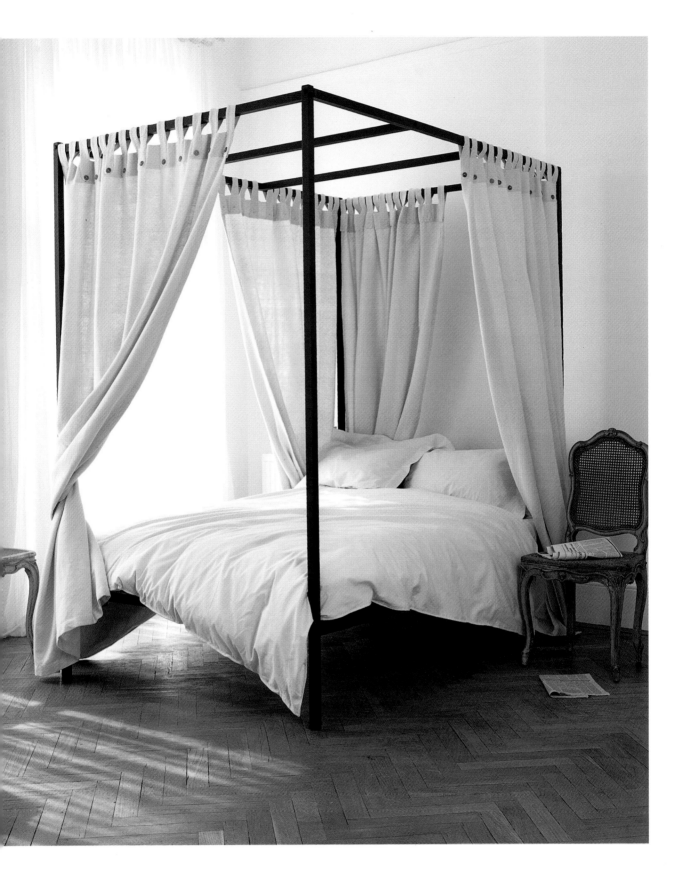

Health considerations are vital in the bedroom, and cutting down on synthetic materials is a good start. Replace items such as polyurethane foam cushions and mattresses, polyester-filled quilts and duvets, polyester-blend sheets, and blankets and throws with non-allergenic natural fibers and fabrics where possible. Not only will you be reducing toxins, but sleeping under cotton, linen or even silk is a pleasure to relish. These natural fibers breathe and help in regulating body temperature.

PVC or vinyl wallpaper also emits chemical vapors so it should be removed and replaced with easily available non-vinyl alternatives, or water-based, naturally-pigmented paint.

Another insidious invader into the bedroom is electromagnetic radiation that is emitted from a range of modern electrical appliances. To reduce it, banish televisions, electric clock-radios, and electric blankets from the bedroom.

An en-suite bathroom, one of the selling-points of many modern homes and apartments, is best kept behind closed doors. Hot baths, steamy showers, damp towels, full-on heating, and poor ventilation all combine to create a heavy, damp atmosphere that will invade the bedroom.

### Choosing the right bed

We are becoming more adventurous with our beds, and standard sewn mattresses and box springs are being replaced in many homes with futons and even water beds. A high-standing bed has two advantages—it allows air to freely circulate under the bed and it is, in the main, much easier for older people to get into and out of.

Unstained wooden headboards and frames are best for obvious holistic reasons, and in feng shui terms, wood can be valued for its neutral effect on ch'i. While wrought iron metal bed ends and frame look beautiful, they act as conductors for electromagnetic radiation.

Whatever bed we choose, it should support the spine while allowing the hips and shoulders to lie comfortably in their natural curvature. A pillow or bolster should support the nape of the neck. This will ensure that the cervical spine remains straight when lying on your side, and curved gently upward when lying on your back.

*Seek out ways of making your bedroom a sanctuary—a health-giving and spirit-rejuvenating place away from it all (RIGHT).*

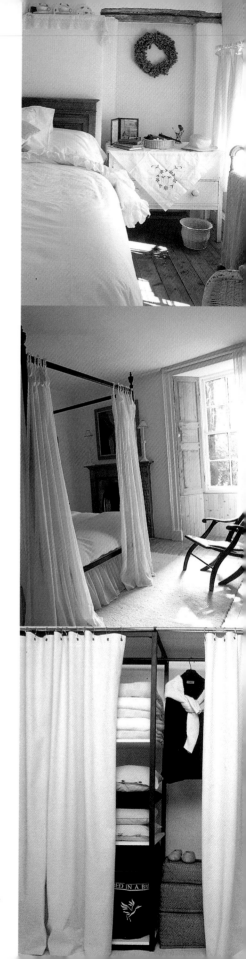

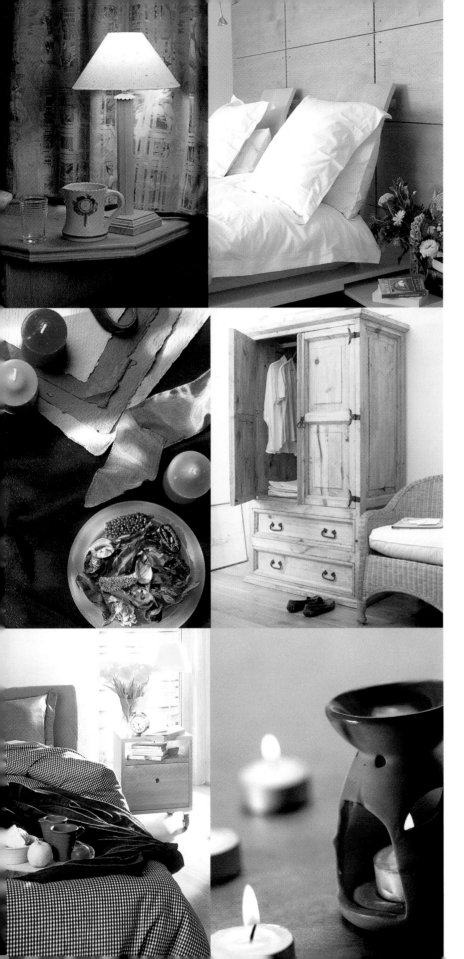

## SENSUOUS
### and calming

Candlelight is wonderful for the bedroom. Blue candles fill the room with a spirit of peace, and green candles can be burnt when someone is ill to aid healing.

Fill the room with calming and evocative scents using scented candles, spray mists or oil essence burners. Other simple methods of introducing scent are to place a few drops of essential on a cold light bulb or onto a candle wick before lighting, or to add six to eight drops of essential oil to a bowl of warm water and place it near a radiator. A novel method is to add an essential oil to the water in a steam iron before pressing bed linen, or add it to the water spray. Never apply oils directly to a fabric— they will stain.

The following will help you to chose the most appropriate oil for your purpose: lavender is calming; rose and geranium will help you gain equilibrium after emotional highs and lows; patchouli or benzoin for a cosy, lazy, and warm atmosphere; frankincense or myrrh if you want to encourage a flagging spirit; and the wafting exotic essences of ylang ylang and sandalwood are unashamedly sensuous.

In the past, how a mattress was made and what it was filled with was surrounded by lore. Feather beds were believed to be effective protection against lightning, dove feathers were very unlucky, and partridge feathers were thought to prevent disease. It was also thought to be important to place beds parallel to visible floorboards to ensure that the energies running through the home would not be impeded by the bed crossing their path.

## FENG SHUI FOR TRANQUILITY

Because we spend so much of our time in bed, the Chinese see the bedroom as an ideal place to get in touch with the natural flow of ch'i energy. This process is not aided if the bedroom doubles as a work room or office. A workstation at the end of a bed not only fills the room with electro-magnetic radiation and an insistent background hum, but it interferes with the flow of ch'i. A bedroom is a sanctuary, not an out-of-town office.

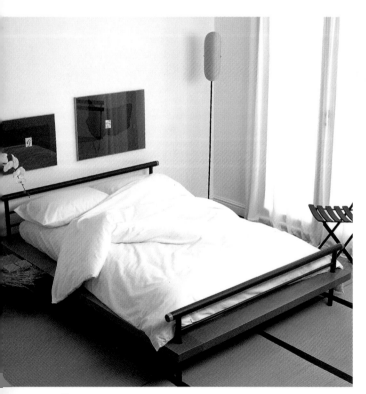

*F*uton, tatami mats, neutral and earth colors, and little distraction from the task of relaxing and rejuvenating.

Light streaming in at dawn is important, so a bedroom located east and south of the center of the home is best. A north-west position is especially recommended for parents as the ch'i energy in this aspect is mature and encourages responsibility, organization, and respect from others. Romance, pleasure, and contentment are emphasized when the bedroom is located in a west segment of the home.

Teenagers, like children, will benefit from the ch'i energy centered in an east or south-east location. The ch'i energy here is directed toward providing a good start in life.

The position of the room also suggests certain color schemes: pink for a northerly bedroom; gray, white, and pink in the north-west; and blues and greens in the east and south. To encourage a peaceful and tranquil atmosphere, colors should be pale rather than strident. Bold colors, patterns or textures are best featured in cushions, throws, and decorative detail.

Anything that will distract from the harmony of the room should be stored away in chests or wardrobes. A calming ch'i energy is fostered if the bedroom is tidied before bedtime,

> *"It's not enough to sleep*
> *—sleep must be organized."*
>
> GEORGE MIKES

and the bed made each morning. Harsh lighting and the jutting edges of furniture will also disturb calming ch'i energy, and destroy the tranquil ambience. Intimacy is symbolized by pairing decorative objects.

Negative ch'i can be countered by concealing sharp corners with round-leafed plants, or softening them with cloths or throws. Ch'i energy can be slowed by using ruched, swagged or draped window dressings, draping a light fabric canopy over the bed, and by hanging rugs on walls. Soft lighting and candlelight with also slow ch'i.

Painting or pictures should be protected with non-reflective glass, rather than reflective glass. Mirrors should be turned to face the wall or covered at night as they will reflect your ch'i while asleep, making it difficult to let go of negative emotions.

**BEDHEAD FACING NORTH**—*the most peaceful and spiritual of all, and it could provide the sleepy solution that an insomniac seeks. Very suitable for older people.*

**BEDHEAD FACING NORTH-WEST**—*suitable for parents and others in positions of authority who need to lead with wisdom. Guarantees a deep and invigorating sleep.*

**BEDHEAD FACING WEST**—*a good sleeping direction for those confident in their career as it can create a sense of contentment. Could aid those who are under stress.*

**BEDHEAD FACING SOUTH-WEST**—*a restful position that may encourage complacency or zealous cautiousness. These could, in turn, lead to instability.*

**BEDHEAD FACING SOUTH**—*sexual and sensual passion will thrive, but so will a passionate temper. Expect poor sleep and strained relationships.*

**BEDHEAD FACING SOUTH-EAST**—*similar to an eastern sleeping direction, but mellower in effect. Auspicious for creativity and communication skills.*

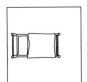

**BEDHEAD FACING EAST**—*a very favorable position, especially for children and teenagers, which urges positive thoughts and actions for the future.*

**BEDHEAD FACING NORTH-EAST**—*sleep in this direction for only limited periods when in need of motivation. It can cause poor sleep interrupted by nightmares.*

## SANDMAN'S *secrets*

✦ IF YOU ARE EXPERIENCING BAD DREAMS OR NEGATIVE FEELINGS, SPRINKLE SALT IN A CIRCLE AROUND THE EDGE OF YOUR BEDROOM AND AROUND YOUR BED.

✦ EUCALYPTUS LEAVES OR CINQUEFOIL PLACED BENEATH THE PILLOW IS SAID TO GUARD YOUR PHYSICAL BODY.

✦ KEEPING A CYCLAMEN OR WAX PLANT IN THE BEDROOM IS BELIEVED TO REFLECT ANY ILL THAT COMES NEAR YOU WHILE ASLEEP, AND A FIR BRANCH HUNG OVER THE BED GUARDS AGAINST SICKNESS OR AIDS SPEEDY RECOVERY.

✦ A STONE WITH A HOLE IN IT, PURSLANE, AND MISTLETOE TWIGS PLACED ON THE BED OR TIED TO A BEDPOST WILL TURN NIGHTMARES INTO BLISSFUL DREAMS.

# 12 child's

## BEDROOM

Whether you are decorating a nursery for a new-born or a bedroom for a toddler or young child, it should be a totally safe living space that is stimulating for play and relaxing for sleep. This room should be declared a toxic material-free zone because young children, like older or infirm people, are the most susceptible to the ill-effects of noxious fumes.

By filling the room with furnishings, fabrics, and toys made from natural materials, and decorating it sympathetically, you can foster in a young child an early respect for nature that will develop into environmental awareness in adulthood.

The first step is to remove synthetic finishes scrupulously, especially from beds and cots, and to replace synthetic flooring, fabrics, and furnishings. Leave wooden surfaces unstained and unpainted, and perfectly smooth so that tiny, sensitive fingers and toes can feel the grain. Make floors comfortable and warm with wool carpet, or with natural-fiber rugs scattered over wood, linoleum, or cork flooring. Sisal and rush floor coverings are very practical, but may abrade tender, young skin. Bedding should be of 100 percent untreated cotton, that is dyed using only natural pigments. Processed, synthetic dyes can cause allergic reactions. Natural materials, like ti-tree bark and cotton, or hypo-allergenic materials should be used for the filling and cover of the mattress.

The second step is to reduce furniture to the minimum so as to free up floor space for games and play. Heavy, sharp-angled pieces of furniture and masses of clutter can cause accidents, but also frustration and confusion.

The third stage is to plan, decorate, and give the room character and atmosphere. Gear your efforts toward making the greatest use of natural light in the play area. Safety considerations may restrict artificial lighting to walls or ceilings, but that does not mean that lighting cannot be used imaginatively. A dimmer switch will cool the lights for a bedtime story, while wall-mounted uplights and downlights can divide the room into areas for play, for drawing, for reading, or for sleeping. Directed light can also be used to highlight a feature, and a colored light bulb can introduce an element of fantasy.

*More than just a cuddly friend, teddy bears (BELOW) are a modern talisman—a totem of good luck.*

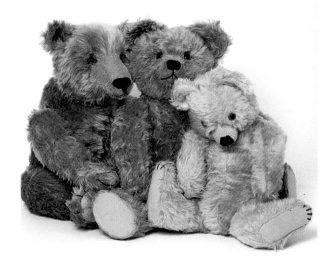

## Stimulating

RELAXING

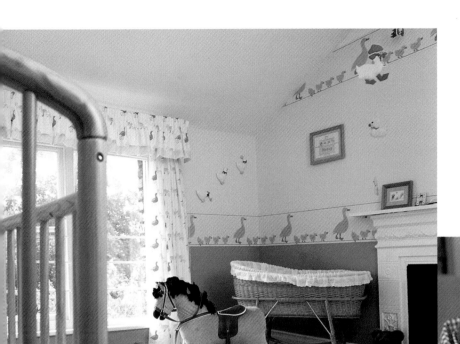

*W*ood and wicker furniture with rounded corners (LEFT) in a spacious, light, and airy bedroom.

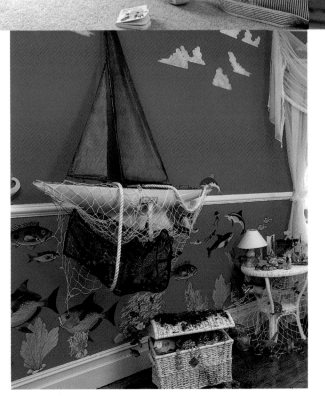

*A* cotton net slung from the keel of the yacht and a cane basket provide storage for toys and beachcombed treasure (RIGHT).

## PROTECTING
*the cradle*

*T*o protect the infant in his cot, every culture has drawn on charms and amulets. In the Greek Orthodox tradition, a blue eye totem is tied to the cot (ABOVE), while the Welsh of Great Britain believe that a knotted length of red ribbon fixed to a child's bed will tie up evil and render it impotent. The bird's nest fern is also believed by some to protect children. Not all charms are rooted in ancient lore—the Theodore Roosevelt-inspired teddy bear of good luck—is a welcome companion in any child's bed.

Storage for toys and all other manner of things is best provided by wood, cane, and bamboo, and by cotton or net bags hung from low wooden pegs. These materials are very practical, yet add something very special. A lidded wooden box becomes a pirate's treasure chest, and cane and wicker baskets his galleon.

It is thought that color has a more profound influence on a child than an adult, untainted as it is by cultural and fashionable associations. It has been found that yellow will promote positive feelings and contribute to the development of thought processes, while a warm—not icy—shade of light blue will relax a child with attention deficit disorder.

Add a few drops of an essential oil to spring water in a spray mist container, or directly onto a cold light bulb (when turned on, heat from the light will warm the oil) to fill the room with relaxing lavender or refreshing orange scents.

### NURSERY FENG SHUI

Favorable situations include east and south-east because they allow the morning sun to energize the room, giving it a youthful, uplifting ch'i that encourages play and creativity. To calm the room for restful sleep, decorate it in soft pastels,

*Bed linen, toys, and storage should be of natural materials. For decorating ideas, look no further than wildlife, the seaside, forest, or garden (RIGHT).*

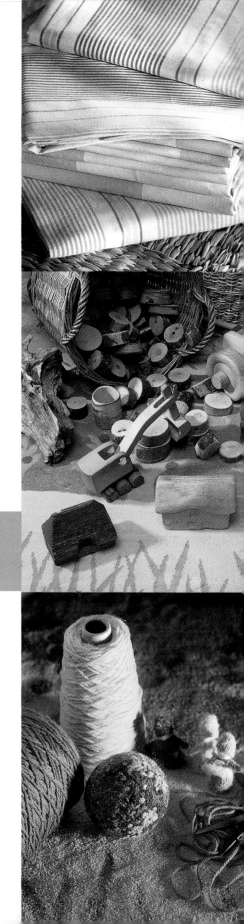

> *"Childhood is measured out by sounds and smells and sights ..."*
> JOHN BETJEMAN

and use star motifs (for fire energy) to quell the tree energy of this location. The afternoon sun will warm a room that is west of the center of the home. This aspect is particularly helpful for children with attention deficit disorder and is supported by a color scheme of calming, soft blues.

A bed placed with its head to the west or north can settle a child who fights sleep, otherwise west or south-east are generally the most favorable. To avoid friction and encourage harmony when two or more children share a room, ensure that their beds are placed in the same direction. Bedheads should not be under a window.

To slow ch'i energy at night, use fabric blinds on the windows and put toys away.

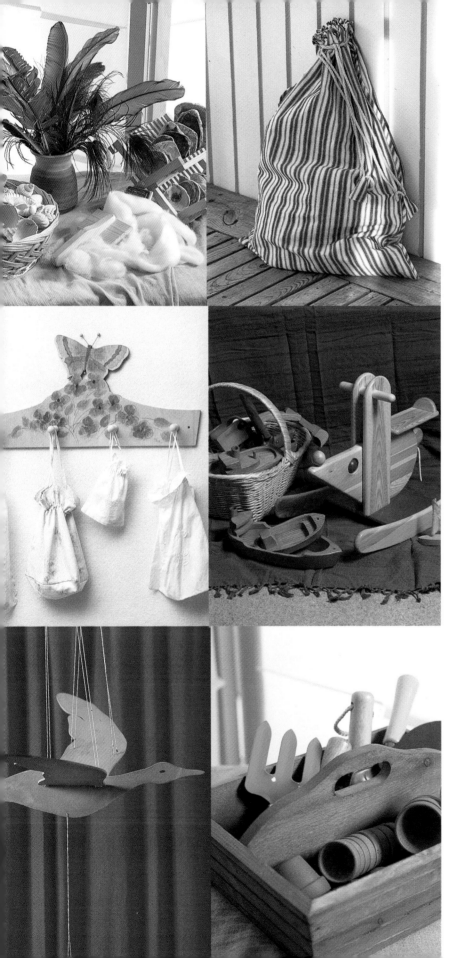

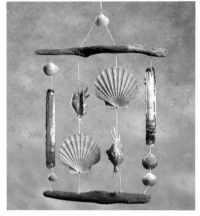

## TOYS *from nature*

*M*obiles—these are more than just decoration: they can be a visual record of a holiday by the sea, or a day spent running through leaves in a fall garden. Lots of carefully balanced horizontal supports are not necessary, and take the project beyond the skill and patience of a child. One or two supports made from twigs, some easily knotted string (or dried grass), and a pile of nature's bounty (ABOVE) are all that's needed. To hang shells that are too hard to make a hole in, glue them securely onto small pieces of card and make the hole in the card. Mobiles hung from the ceiling can be arousing or relaxing, depending on the colors and materials used, but do not hang mobiles directly over a bed.

Building blocks—create a highly individual collection from off-cuts of wood left over from do-it-yourself projects or begged from a timber yard, and twigs, bark and driftwood—the more unusual the shape, the better. Clean and then dry the pieces of wood in an airing cupboard or on a warm, dry window ledge before sanding them. The blocks can be colored using natural stains or rubbed with beeswax.

# bathroom

BATHROOM

Nineteenth-century Western notions about bathing as a necessary evil, rather than a pleasure, are gradually being replaced with altogether more Eastern concepts. In the East, bathing is a ritual that involves physical and psychological cleansing and relaxation. It is not the job of one minute, but a pleasure to be lingered over, often in the company of others. Little wonder, then, that an Eastern bathroom looks full of promise, in comparison to the function-over-fun Western equivalent where few of us want to dwell, let alone entertain. But things are changing, and changing in a way that is holistic.

A good place to start is by looking at a Japanese bathing area. For even though the ancient Greeks and Romans, and the Scandinavians, had the right idea about bubbling spas and hot tubs, the Japanese made bathing an art.

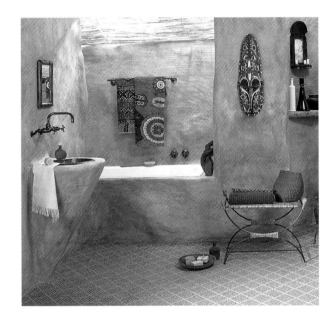

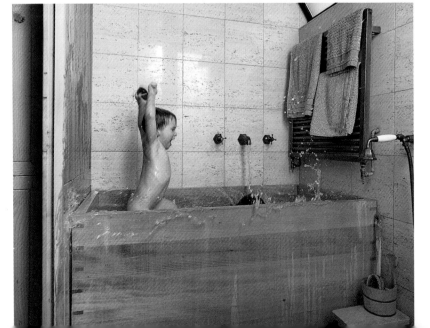

*Bathrooms can be pleasing to the eye and functional. It is purely personal taste that determines its style (ABOVE AND RIGHT).*

*A wooden Japanese-style bath (LEFT) deeper but smaller than a modern Western bath. Before getting into the bath you have a cleansing shower.*

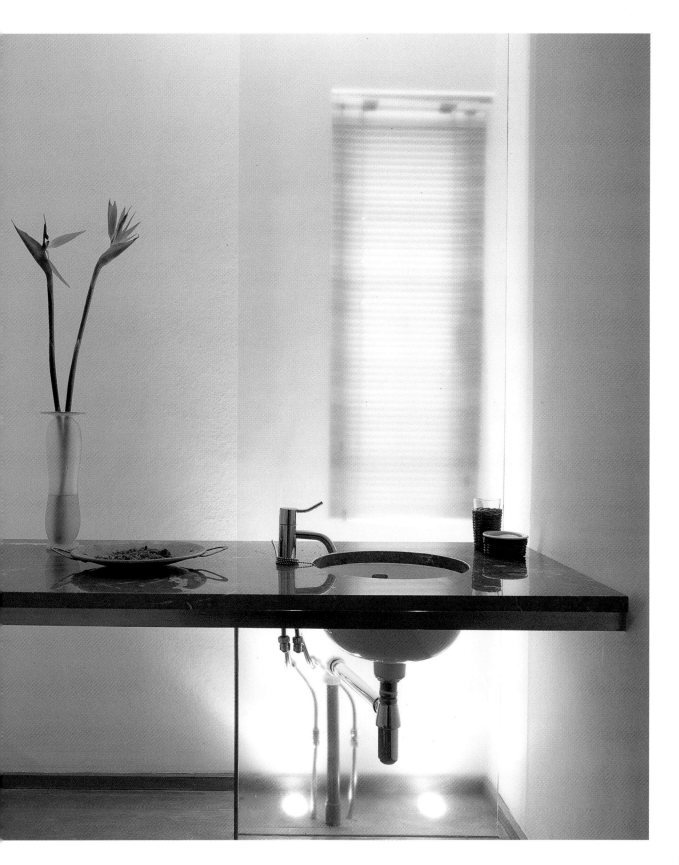

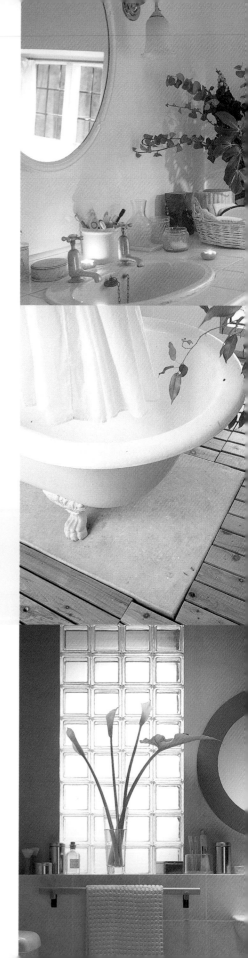

In a traditional Japanese home, the bathing area was made as large as possible, and was afforded equal decorating and design zeal as any other room. Ventilation, natural light, aspect, color, texture, smell, and comfort were paramount, but so was water and energy conservation.

To change the water in the bath for each new bather was considered wasteful, so bathers would shower first, thereby separating bathing for hygiene and bathing for relaxation. Since Japanese baths are deeper and have a smaller surface area, they remain warmer for longer. Heat loss is further reduced by covering the bath.

The calming atmosphere of an Eastern bathing area is guaranteed by the plentiful use of natural materials—unstained wood, bamboo, wicker, cane, clay tiles, stone, plaster, untreated cork, mulberry paper screens—and luxurious natural accessories like loofahs, sisal friction gloves, sea sponges, cotton towels, essences and oils, herbal soaps, plants, and serene flower arrangements.

To go totally Japanese in your bathroom may be impossible, but some adjustments can be realised in even the

*The calming atmosphere of an Eastern bathing area is guaranteed by the plentiful use of natural materials.*

smallest bathroom. Rubber mats, plastic or nylon shower curtains, plastic laundry basket, and synthetic bath accessories can be replaced with wooden mats, natural fabrics, a wicker laundry basket, and totally natural shampoos, soaps, and oils.

Conserve water and energy by fitting low-flow taps, half-flush toilet cisterns, water temperature limiters, and opt for showers rather than baths. Substitute an automatic extractor fan that whines on forever for a manual one that is operated by a switch or cord, thereby improving natural ventilation. Increase the amount of natural light entering, and fill the bathroom with plants.

In such a rejuvenated environment, bathing is lingered over and the cleansing is more than skin deep.

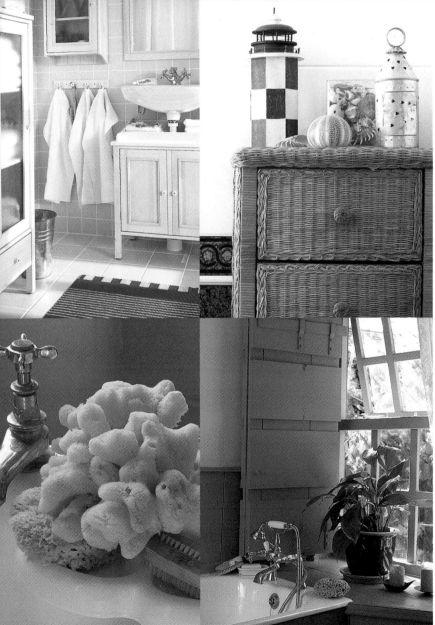

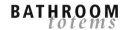

# BATHROOM
*totems*

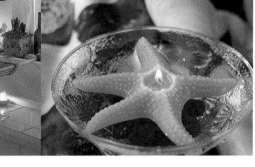

*T*he idea that people, places, events, and even rooms have spirit guides, or totems, is common in many cultures. A totem can, imbue a room with a specific energy.

✦ TOTEMS STRONGLY ASSOCIATED WITH THE BATHROOM INCLUDE DOLPHINS, WHALES, FISH, SEALS, TURTLES, AND FROGS, THOUGH MANY OTHER WATER CREATURES CAN ALSO BE SIGNIFICANT. A PLASTER OR PORCELAIN MODEL, PICTURE, OR PATTERN INCORPORATING ONE OR MORE OF THESE TOTEMS WILL BRING THE SPIRIT OF WATER, AND THE ENERGIES OF LIFE AND NATURE INTO THE BATHROOM.

*FROM TOP, LEFT TO RIGHT: Pale colors; a vase of leafy foliage, and smooth, rounded surfaces under flickering candle light; glass brick bath of Japanese dimensions; candle power; bath set on a stone slab in the middle of a wood floor; wood cabinets, towels, and rug to help deaden sound; cane chest of drawers; serene flower arrangement; natural bathing companions—sea sponges; a healthy bathroom full of fresh air and natural light.*

# HOMEMADE
*naturally*

### Citrus bath oil

*In a glass bottle, mix ⅓ cup avocado or almond base oil with 1 tablespoon lemon essential oil, 2 teaspoons orange essential oil, and 1 teaspoon lime essential oil. Seal and store the mixture for two weeks. Add 1 tablespoon of the oil to a bath of warm water.*

*Healthy, thriving plants help counteract the humid and damp atmosphere of a bathroom, even a well ventilated one like this (RIGHT).*

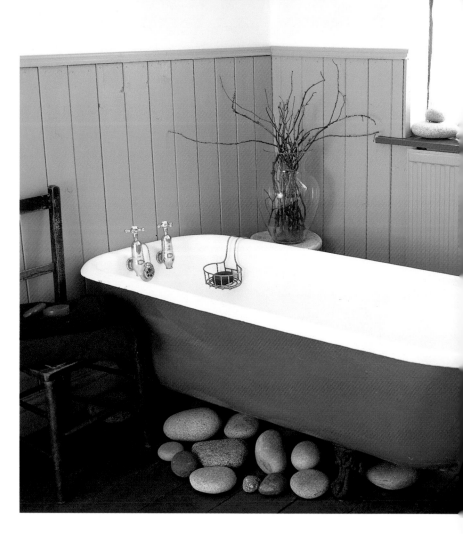

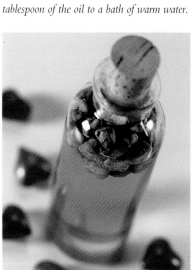

### Rosemary water

*Add 1 lb fresh herbs and 8 oz dried herbs to a saucepan containing 1 pt spring water. Bring the mixture gently to a boil, then cover and simmer for 10 minutes. Allow to cool before straining and reserving the liquid. Pour the liquid into a 2 pt bottle and add ½ cup vodka. Pour ¼ pt of the rosemary water into a warm bath.*

### Sunrise pick-me-up

*To combat fatigue, add three drops thyme oil, two drops rosemary oil, and one drop lavender oil to a morning bath.*

### Sunset soother

*Add four drops lavender oil and two drops bergamot to an evening bath.*

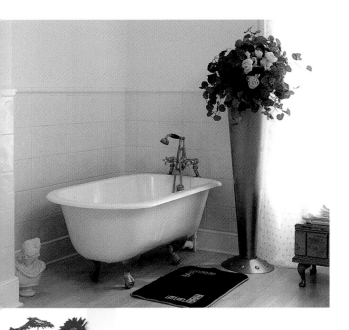

The warmth of the bathroom will accentuate the scent of natural materials, but this can be complemented by essential oils and aromatherapy candles. Peppermint and pine oils are stimulating, cleansing, and refreshing; while sensuous heavens beckon with the scents of rose or ylang ylang.

### FENG SHUI IN THE BATHROOM

The most favorable location is east or south-east of the center of the home, away from a staircase, dining room, and kitchen, and not opposite the main door. Auspicious color schemes in these situations are cream and off-white with green and dark blue accessories. Introduce irregular patterns, possibly with water as a theme, wherever possible.

The flooring and wall surfaces should be smooth so as not to scatter ch'i, so wood, marble, and granite surfaces are preferred to tiled or mosaic ones. To counter the effects of such surfaces, introduce earth elements like terracotta, stones, and natural fibers.

*The bedroom that became a spacious and gracious bathroom (ABOVE) and (BELOW) a low wall separates the toilet from the bath.*

As water is the main element, damp or wet surfaces and a humid atmosphere can cause ch'i to stagnate. Counter this with plentiful natural light, ventilation, and plants. Such

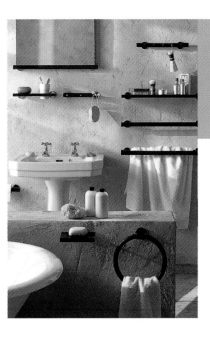

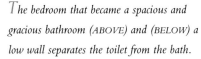

> *"The way to health is to have an aromatic bath and scented massage every day."*
>
> **H I P P O C R A T E S**

remedies are not possible in windowless en suite bathrooms so it is crucial that walls are painted with water-based, microporous paints, and that timber and cork on walls or floors are left unsealed. Animate ch'i in such bathrooms with bright artificial lighting, shiny surfaces, chrome fixtures, and mirrors fixed to adjoining walls.

A separate toilet is also desirable, since toilets drain ch'i downward and exacerbate the problems of stagnation. A satisfactory compromise is to screen the toilet from the rest of the bathroom, and always ensure the toilet seat is down lest you lose not only ch'i energy but also, according to feng shui, money!

*A link to a river flowing over stones is clearly the achieved aim in this blue and white bathroom (LEFT).*

# 14 a retreat

A RETREAT

A retreat—a place of escape—will offer all who live in the home a space in which to seek healing, rest, and inspiration. It does not matter if it is a box room, part of a converted attic or an outbuilding, what is important is that it should be uncompromisingly conducive to quiet activities.

To be assured of privacy and uninterrupted solitude, you may have to entreat others in the home to agree to honor the sanctity of the retreat. This will be more easily achieved if they understand that they, too, can use the room for its intended purpose.

*"Meditation here. May think down hours to moments ...And Learning grow wiser without his Books."*

WILLIAM COWPER

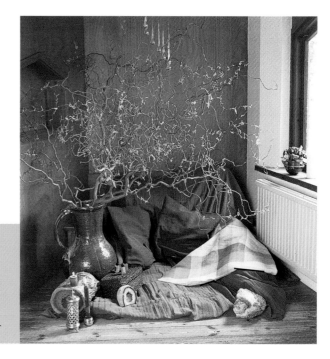

The atmosphere you want to promote is one of intimacy, safety, warmth, and tranquility. But however you achieve this atmosphere, the key is simplicity and the principle is this: an empty space makes it easier to empty the mind.

Furniture should be minimal. So rather than approaching it as a decorating project, start using the room when it contains nothing more than a chair, cushions or a yoga mat. Then you will know exactly what is necessary, rather than what would look good. It might be that you need to warm the room with soft rugs in warm colors, or include something inspirational that will provide a focus for meditation. Fussy patterns will distract, so seek out plain fabrics in subdued colors.

*A retreat takes no specific form, it is an area—large or small—that reflects your needs. In this retreat (ABOVE), curly willow stems define this area as separate to the rest of the room.*

## Meditation

TRANQUILITY

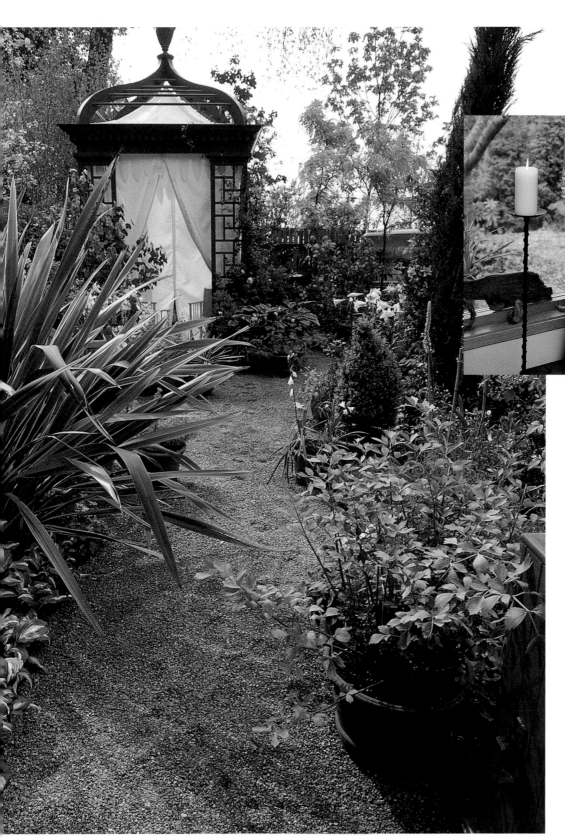

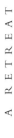

*If your retreat looks onto a garden (ABOVE), use it as a focus for your meditation.*

*An idylic summer house screened by plants and cotton curtains and scented by flowers doubles as an retreat (LEFT).*

# CREATING THE
## *right atmosphere*

- ✦ A DISH OF WATER OR A QUARTZ CRYSTAL WILL BRING A SENSE OF LOVE, CONTENTMENT, AND SPIRITUALITY TO A RETREAT.

- ✦ SCENT THE ROOM WITH ONE DROP FRANKINCENSE AND FOUR DROPS OF SANDALWOOD ADDED TO A SPRAY MIST CONTAINER FILLED WITH PURIFIED WATER. THE SOPORIFIC EFFECT OF THESE ESSENTIAL OILS WILL CALM, RELEASE FEAR, AND REDUCE STRESS.

- ✦ INCENSE, TOO, IS EXCELLENT IN A RETREAT ROOM. TRY, FOR EXAMPLE, ALMOND FOR WISDOM, AND CINNAMON FOR SPIRITUALITY, HEALING, AND PROTECTION.

- ✦ BLUE, PURPLE OR WHITE CANDLES ARE IDEAL FOR A MEDITATION ROOM.

- ✦ FINE TUNE THE SUBTLE ENERGIES WITH HOMEOPATHIC AND BACH FLOWER REMEDIES.

- ✦ IF MUSIC CAN SOOTHE THE SAVAGE BREAST, THEN IT MOST PROBABLY HAS A PLACE IN A RETREAT. DO NOT CONFINE YOURSELF TO FAVORITES, BUT LOOK ALSO AT RECORDINGS OF NATURAL SOUNDS. IT MAY BE THAT ALL YOU NEED TO SET THE TONE IN YOUR RETREAT, IS THE METALLIC DING OF A SMALL BELL.

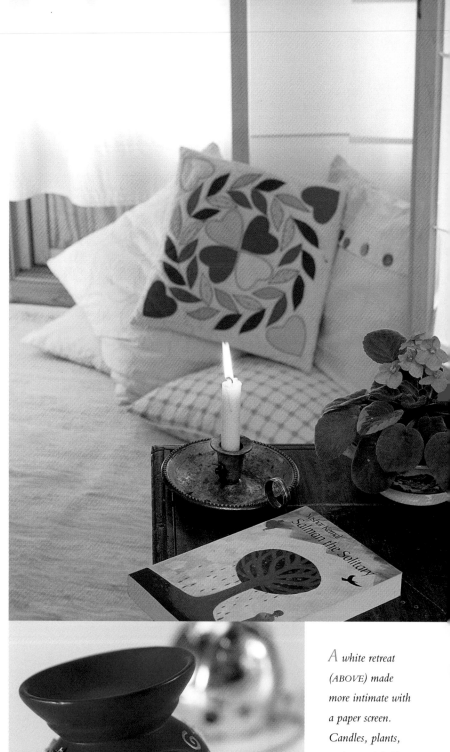

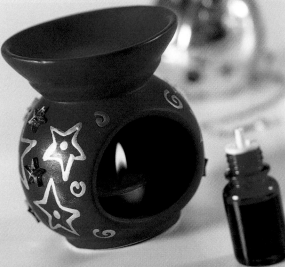

*A white retreat (ABOVE) made more intimate with a paper screen. Candles, plants, and essential oils are used to create a relaxing, healing atmosphere.*

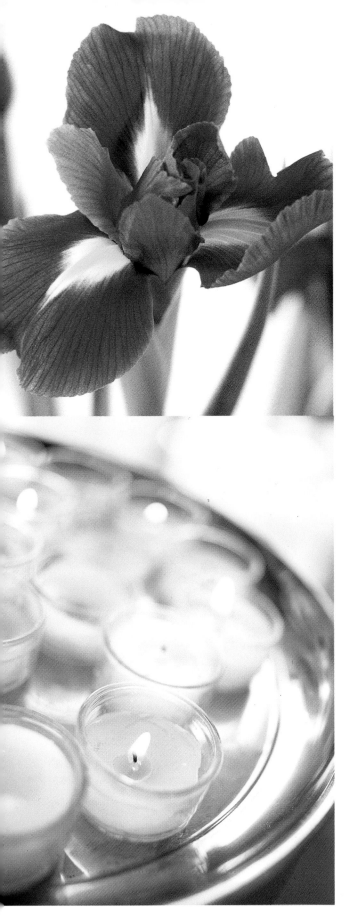

*A simple bowl of pebbles (RIGHT) can provide a focus for meditation—their colors are harmonious, their texture hypnotic, and they remind you of nature's endurance and strength.*

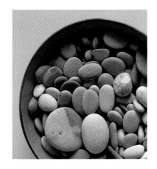

# Sanctity

## INTIMACY

Lighting should be gentle and unobtrusive, and window dressings used to filter harsh sunlight and to provide total privacy. If your retreat is blessed with a beautiful view, do not obscure it, but use it in the process of relaxing.

An all-white room feels clean and clear, and this in turn can help you clear your mind and to relax profoundly. Other colors that promote meditation are blue and purple. Blue creates an atmosphere of serenity and truth, and purple, psychic awareness and intuition. These colors are suggestions only—you must follow your own instincts and choose a color scheme that feels right for you.

For those who enjoy massage, yoga or other Eastern forms of exercise, a therapy room may be an ideal retreat. Your therapy room will need a massage table or mat, a simple but pleasing wooden box for essential oils and base oils, fluffy cotton towels, or a yoga mat. Create the calming atmosphere as you would for a meditation room, but a pot plant or fresh flowers can be a pleasing addition.

There is a sense in which, whatever your religious beliefs, a retreat should be dedicated to its purpose, or blessed, before you begin to use it. You may therefore wish to offer a simple prayer or light a votive candle as a personal gesture.

# 15 plants for

## PLEASURE AND BOUNTY

Few homes are without a carefully tended windowbox, an array of pot plants, or a vase of cut flowers; and for those with a garden the pleasure of the company of nature's bounty is simply multiplied many times. We have, as have generations before us, a love of plants. Even the most hardened individual cannot fail to be moved in some way by dew-drop glistening petals, the scent of jasmine or honeysuckle, the rustle of leaves overhead, or the tickle of soft grass underfoot. The smell, texture, color, and look of plants, in all their guises, play to all our senses and profoundly affect us, while tending them satisfies deep psychological needs.

### Indoor friends

Plants, as living things, are very special decorative objects. Because they constantly photosynthesize carbon dioxide into carbohydrates and oxygen, plants create a fresher, more energizing atmosphere. They also help to counteract the effects of electrical radiation, and to balance humidity. In an office or study, peace lilies or spider plants set in a tray of damp peat or compost, will do wonders for air quality. In return for their natural benevolence though, plants need to be cared for and placed in appropriate positions.

According to feng shui, plants and even cut flowers generate their own flow of ch'i energy, but if left to wilt or languish in stagnant water they affect ch'i negatively. The energy of a plant is determined by its color and shape. The brilliant blue of the cornflower or delphinium is providential for travel and communication, and the fringed petals of the carnation are linked to romance. Leaf shape is also

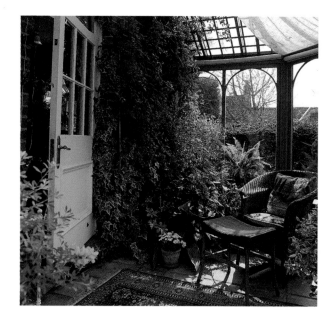

*The tranquil atmosphere of these two very different rooms (ABOVE AND RIGHT) is created by well-tended and carefully chosen plants.*

influential: pointed, stiff leaves help ch'i move more quickly, and rounded, soft leaves calm ch'i. An ivy, allowed to trail over a sharp corner, prevents the flow of ch'i being cut; but to deter burglars, place a spiky cactus on a window ledge.

Plant aromas have a subtle effect on our emotions, so fresh herbs in the kitchen, and a pot of lavender in the living room, for example, can be used to create different moods. Give plants a chance to release their scent by placing them where your hand or legs can gently brush against them, or where their scent will be picked up on a breeze and carried through the home.

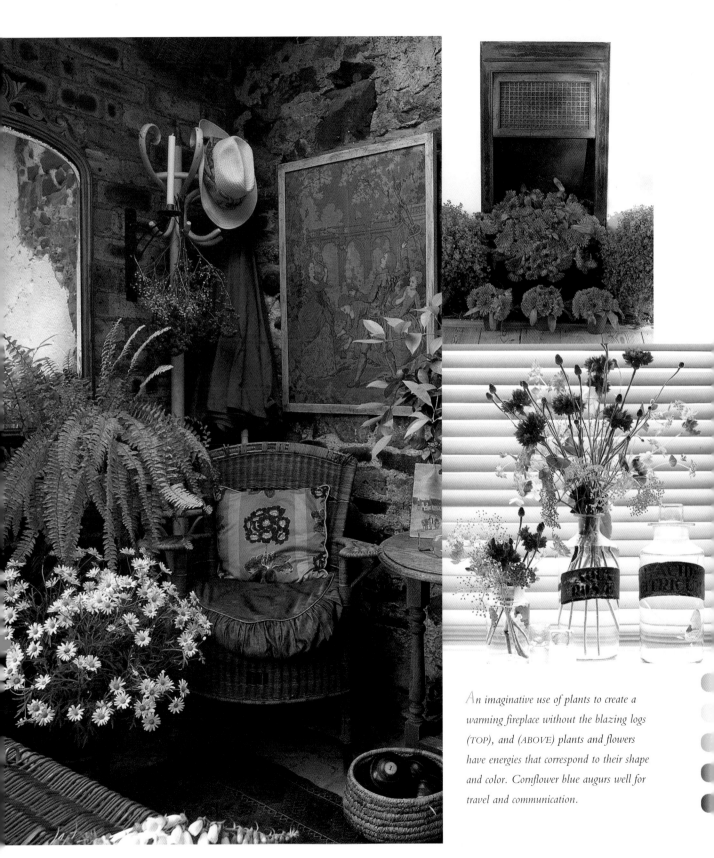

*An imaginative use of plants to create a warming fireplace without the blazing logs (TOP), and (ABOVE) plants and flowers have energies that correspond to their shape and color. Cornflower blue augurs well for travel and communication.*

## The sensual and spiritual garden

Whether your garden reflects the formal style of a grand house with rolling lawns and immaculate flower beds, or a cottage garden full of vegetables, fruit trees, herbaceous borders, and rose-covered arbors, a more holistic effect can be created by incorporating elements that foster spirituality and appeal to all the senses.

Eastern cultures have always seen gardens as spiritual places that provide oases of peace. The Japanese garden, influenced by the Shinto faith, is a good example of this. Subtle earth tones dominate, and the continuity of life is represented by seasonal color changes in trees and shrubs. The Chinese use their gardens as a way of symbolically representing nature's crucial elements of springs, rivers, mountains, and rock. At first glance, your garden may appear devoid of any exotic influence, but if you have chrysanthemums, peonies, camellias, hostas, or clematis growing, then East and West have met. These plants and many others originated in Japan and China.

*A wealth of ideas (RIGHT) that will bring sound, texture, color, scent, and spirituality into your garden*

> *"Very much like painting or sculpture, gardening is a means of giving physical, sensory form to emotional or spiritual matters."*
>
> MARC P. KEANE

Spiritual dimensions can be achieved with wind chimes, crystals, man-made and natural rock sculptures, and water features. Heighten sensual feedback with highly scented plants, paying particular attention to those plants whose scent is strongest at different times of the day. Jasmine, night-scented stock, and nicotiana (tobacco plant) have heady evening perfumes, while lavender and honeysuckle emit their scents all day long. Choose plants in colors that you find uplifting, and textures that excite—delicate ferns, feathery grasses and catkins, wiry tendrils, silky smooth or coarse stems, velvety leaves. To drown out unwanted noise—or at least to distract you from it—include a tinkling water fountain or plants, like bamboo, poplar, and reeds, that will make lovely swooshing noises in the wind.

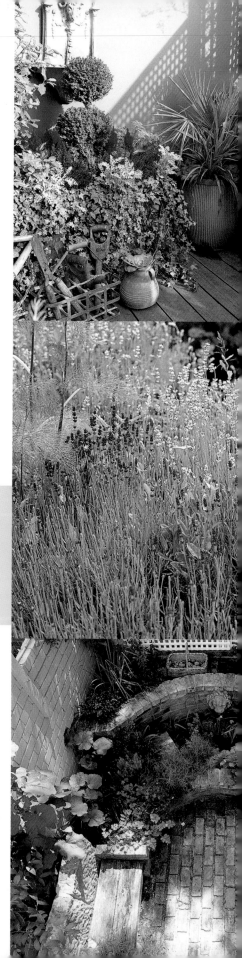

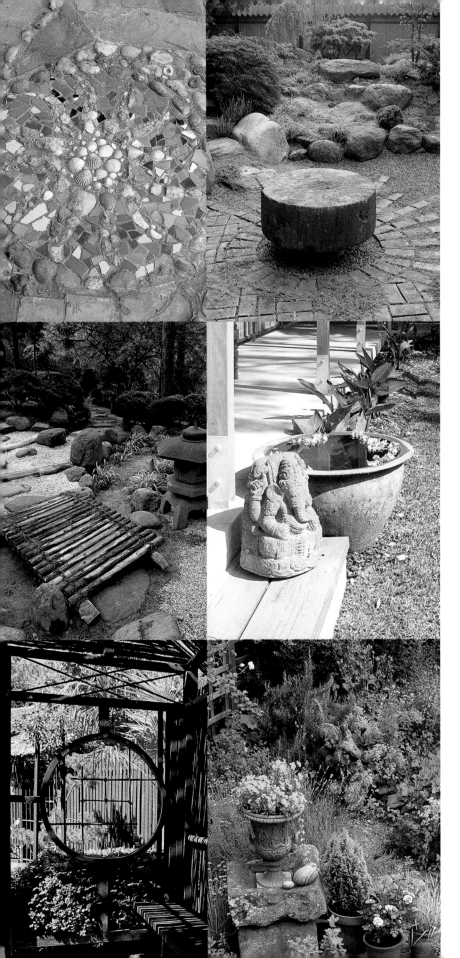

## THE POWER
### *of trees*

*W*e are all attracted to trees and hugging them is not unknown—even the heir to the British throne, Prince Charles, has admitted to the practice. To stand beside a towering sequoia or beech tree that is hundreds of years old fills us with a sense of permanence and security, and not a little humility. In shaman traditions, trees are doors between this world and other worlds, and stand guard on the threshold between the two. Trees are a source of healing and a focus for meditation in many cultures. To have a tree in your garden is a privilege and a pleasure that outlasts the seasons.

## HOMEMADE
### *pesticides*

*T*o control slugs—boil dry wormwood leaves in water to cover, then strain. Dilute the strained liquid with water in the ratio of one part wormwood tea to five parts water. Spray onto the plant.

To control aphids—boil up tomato leaves and stems in water for five minutes. Strain, and when the reserved liquid is cool pour it into a spray mist container and use immediately. Use frequently and apply generously to keep aphids at bay.

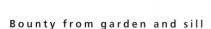

### Bounty from garden and sill

There is something inherently satisfying about growing your own food, even if it is only a pot of chives on a windowsill. The care and investment you have made in the plant translates into better-tasting food. The seasonal nature of produce is now so easily forgotten with supermarkets stocking just about everything imaginable year-round. Many children do not appreciate that strawberries and raspberries, for example, were once summer time treats only. When you grow your own vegetables and fruits you are re-acquainted with the cycles of nature and can enjoy foods when they are at their best—apples in the fall, sprouts in winter, crisp lettuces in late spring.

As more and more people have come to recognize the health hazards of chemical fertilizers and pesticides, home-grown and organically produced food has become more popular. Not everyone has the time, space or dedication to become self-sufficient. The key is to do as much as you can and to enjoy the experience. Your efforts may be restricted to herbs growing in a windowbox or on a windowsill, or to pots of tomatoes, beans, and strawberries on a balcony. A do-it-yourself enthusiast could build a window frame greenhouse onto a sun-drenched window.

Successful organic gardening relies on cultivating the soil with natural minerals and organic fertilizers that actually create soil. The current thinking in most commercial ventures is to stimulate soil for greater productivity with the zealous addition of chemicals and pesticides. These chemicals also eventually destroy the soil. Even plant-based pesticides should be used with caution. Derris dust, which is almost synonymous with growing tomatoes, can accumulate in the body, while pyrethrum may cause eye problems.

Those new to organic gardening worry about being able to control insect pests without the help of chemical pesticides. In fact, plants that are grown on good organic soil boosted by kitchen and garden compost tend to suffer less from insects and disease. Companion planting many also help.

Companion planting involves selecting and positioning plants so that they benefit from those plants around them. Some plants, for example, exude substances from their roots that will destroy a pest or soil-induced disease in another plant. Companion planting also encourages a wide variety of insects to the site, so that one species of insect cannot dominate. This is an example of how companion planting can work: citrus trees attract, among other insects, aphids but if you plant broad beans nearby, the broad bean will attract the aphid as well as enrich the soil with its stores of nitrogen. Other favorable and flowering pairings are: strawberries and beans, and tomatoes and garlic. Stifle weeds under ground-hugging camomile and lemon. The lemon thyme, as will any lemon-scented plant, will control mosquitoes. Companion planting is a vast topic, and your local plantsman will be able to help.

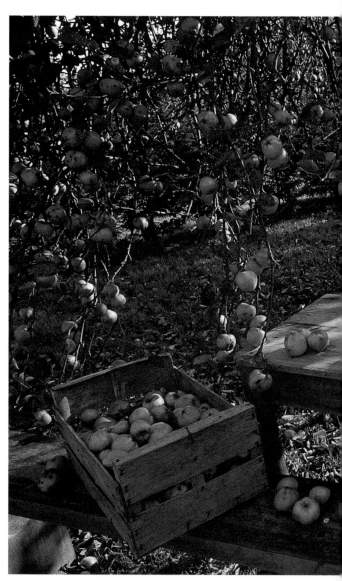

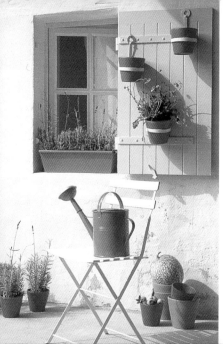

*Whether gardening pots of herbs on the sill or porch (LEFT) or an orchard of fruiting trees (BELOW), producing food for your table intimately re-acquaints you with the cycles of nature.*

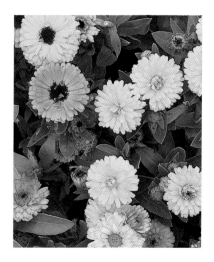

## THE RECYCLING
*chain*

*F*irst you need a compost bin made from wood or bricks. Its size is purely dependent on the size of your garden, but it should be positioned as far away from the home as possible, yet central to make distribution of the compost over the garden less of a chore. To make it easy to dig the compost out of the bin, the front panel should be removable. A brick compost bin needs to be constructed with plenty of openings for ventilation.

Next you need material to compost. Pile up garden waste—weeds, grass clippings, leaves and so on—in front of the bin, and for every bucket of kitchen waste added to the bin, cover it with a generous layer of garden waste to deter birds and dogs. To set off the process, pour a bucket of "household liquid activator" (one part urine to three parts water), or a commercial equivalent, over the compost. The compost will reach a temperature of 160°–170°F within the first 10 days. The growth of fungi inside the compost will then cause the temperature to drop. A compost set off in the summer will be ready for use in the fall, and one started over fall and winter will be ripe for spring.

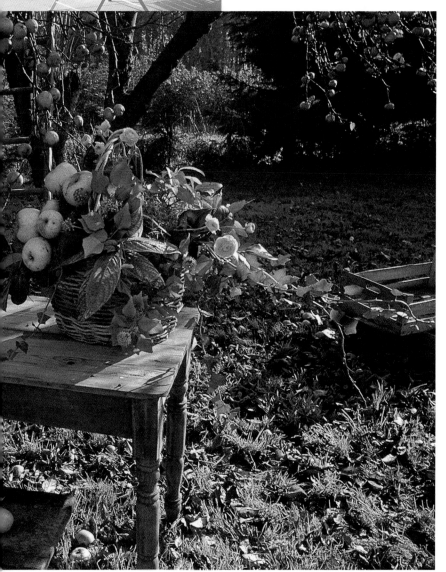

# CHAPTER 16

# *living*

## HOLISTICALLY

In the past, the freedom to choose a particular way of life was a privilege afforded to very few people. For most, life was a struggle, and success measured by the ability to satisfy the basic human needs of warmth, shelter, and sustenance. Today, in wealthier parts of the world at least, those needs being met means that people have time to look at ways of improving the quality of their lives and introducing more balance between work and play.

> *Make tomorrow better
> by living well today.*

### Managing time holistically

To have the time to fulfill all the different areas of your life, without getting stressed in the process, is managing time holistically. You achieve whatever you choose to achieve in a day, and what is not accomplished is quite calmly set aside for tackling another day.

The trick lies in understanding your values (those things that you believe to be worthwhile) and knowing your goals (the ends toward which effort or ambition is directed). When considering your values you must take into account your whole being—the physical, psychological, emotional, social, and spiritual. Armed with this knowledge you can then set realistic priorities—one of which will be managing your health—and make flexible plans.

On a day-to-day level, you need to get to know yourself. When, for example, is your best time? Are you an early bird or night owl? Use your own natural rhythms to get the best out of your day; work when you work best, rest when sleepy and tired. Forget standard time constraints, and develop a personal sense of time that works for you.

### The elements of an holistic day

To satisfy your whole being you should include at least one activity from each of the following in your holistic day plan:

✦ Physical—change your routine so that you walk more; eat raw fruit and vegetables at one meal; or have an early night after a relaxing bath.

✦ Psychological—erase worry from your mind and think about something totally positive and uplifting for five minutes every day; before starting work—whether that be in an office or in the kitchen—clear a space so that you can start afresh; or do a stress breaking exercise.

✦ Emotional—see how many times you smile in a day, and then do it more often; hug someone you love; and to release tension, do as Liza Minnelli did in *Cabaret*—try shouting while a train crosses a railway bridge above you.

✦ Social—contact a friend or relative for a chat; play a sport or a game alone or in company; or do something for someone else—it feels surprisingly good.

✦ Spiritual—light a candle for someone who is important to you, and while the candle burns, wish them well; take inspiration from a thing of beauty; or take stock of the good things in your life.

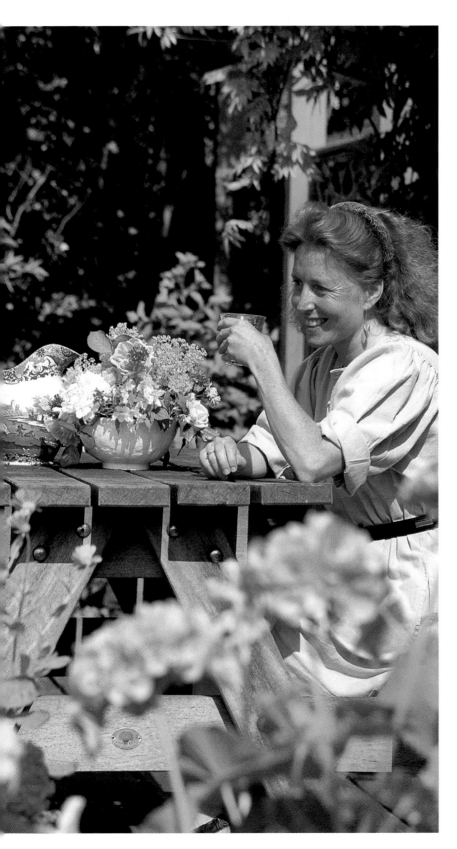

## DOWNSHIFTING
### *stress*

*T*he fewer things you must do in life, the fewer things you own, manage or are responsible for, the fewer are the stresses upon you. Tough words in a materialistic world, but true nonetheless.

The 1980s saw an alarming increase in consumerism, but by the 1990s many of us were either shopped-out or ready for a change. That change came to be known as downshifting. People looked at the long hours they worked; the time not spent with their children, partners, friends, and family; and health- and life- strengthening activities that they were missing—and they realised they were simply not enjoying themselves. Some people decided to simplify their lives, get rid of what they did not need, work out how much money they really needed, and earn it in the least stressful, fairest, and ecologically sound way possible. Some people chose to move away from urban areas, while others remained but changed their lifestyle to a less hectic, less materialistic one. Downshifting in the United States is affecting between five and ten percent of the workforce. In Britain signs of a similar trend are emerging. One poll recently found that 64 percent of full-time workers would give up their current jobs if they could afford to.

*F*inding the time to stop, relax, and take stock of the good things in your life is an important part of living holistically.

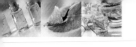

# PET *companions*

*I*n the past, animals were kept for their usefulness—as sources of food and raw materials, and as beasts of burden. But the notion that animals can also be beneficial companions has only recently been explored. In nursing homes, the presence of a pet improves the sense of well-being among both staff and patients. In one study, it was noted that an elderly man spoke his first coherent sentence for 26 years as a result of his interactions with the nursing home's resident dog.

But healthy adults and children also benefit. Children derive comfort from soft objects such as stuffed toys, and family pets may fulfill a similar role. Pets become confidants and friends, and provide a way to approach difficult subjects such as sex and death. In adulthood, pets offer other unexpected benefits. For example, survival after a heart attack is significantly higher among pet owners, due to the pets' calming effect. Moreover, heart rate and blood pressure reduce while stroking and interacting with animals. Elderly people with pets, for example, receive more spontaneous visits from friends and family, and owners talk of the personal fulfillment they feel from caring for their animals.

However, there are health risks, including infection and allergic reactions, associated with keeping pets that should not be underestimated.

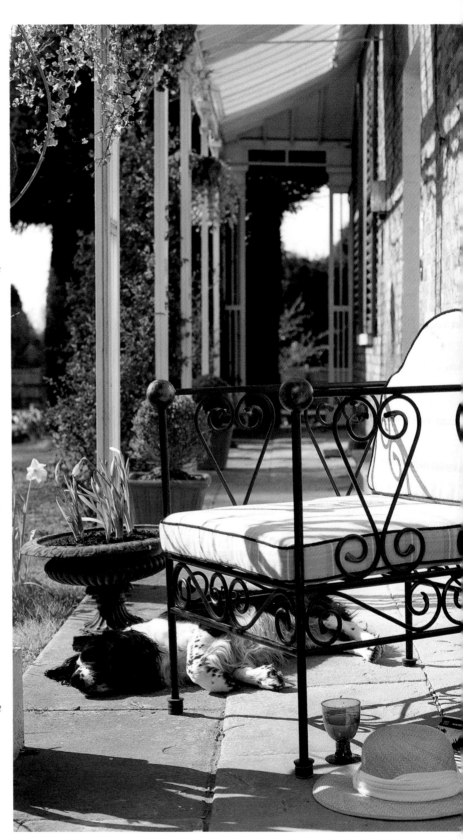

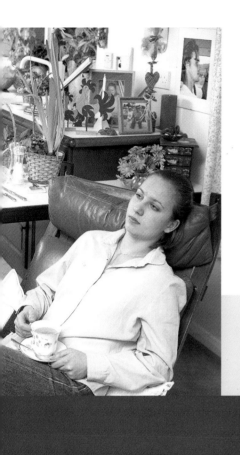

*Give yourself five minutes time-out during the day (LEFT) and why not spend an evening counting stars (BELOW).*

## Stress

Stress is caused by how you assess an event and by how you then respond to that assessment. If you think "So what!" and mean it, there is no adverse stress, but if you react differently then stress steps in, steps up, and can take over.

The physiological link between illness and stress arises from your reaction to threats. This "fight or flight" reaction provokes a dramatic increase in adrenal hormones and catecholamines such as cortisol and adrenaline. As the levels of adrenaline rise, your heart beat accelerates, blood pressure rises, and breathing becomes more rapid. Rises in cortisol levels act as an anti-inflammatory agent, limiting inflammation at the site of any injury that has occurred.

> *"Let all your things have their places. Let each part of your business have its time"*
>
> ### BENJAMIN FRANKLIN

This is a natural and important reaction to danger that prepares you so that you can respond to the threat. However, it also occurs as a reaction to stressful events, and this is where the issue of stress taking over comes in. The buzz of a challenge at work, for example, can be positive and rewarding. However, repeated provocation of these hormones, for example because we have too much work with too many urgent problems to solve, exerts a great strain on your cardiovascular and immune system. Stress then becomes dangerous and can have a negative effect on health.

We all have different ways of coping with stress. Some of us take a rational route—making lists, seeking help, delegating. Others have a more emotional response, and burst into floods of tears or angry outbursts. There are also the ostriches who block out the problem, or deny there is one. The lucky ones are those who can see themselves as independent of the problem.

While emotional and avoidance coping strategies may give immediate relief, they are ultimately unhelpful. In the long term we become increasingly overwhelmed, or unable to maintain a head in the sand attitude. Developing more rational and detached coping strategies, however, can have long term benefits. A key element in managing stress is communication. Stress causes poor communication, which in turn causes more stress—a damaging vicious circle. Communication is the medium through which stress is expressed, so it can also be a way of alleviating it. Improving our communication skills makes the expression of emotion easier, helping others to know how we feel. It is also true that being able to express how we feel is itself a coping mechanism, allowing us to externalize, rather than bottle up, our feelings.

*A perfect image of great symbolism (BELOW) that you could use as a focus for meditation.*

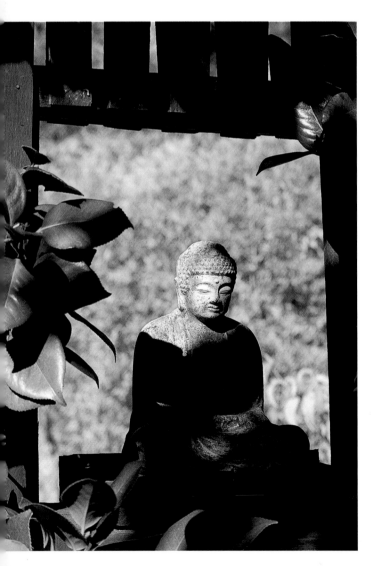

## Breaking the stress spiral

### Relaxation

The simplest way of beginning to relax is by becoming aware of the effect tension has on our body, and practicing "stopping." When you become aware of being caught in a stressful spiral, just stop and become aware of your body. You will probably find that your shoulders are raised, your face frowning and your stomach tense. Try relaxing by letting all the tension go from your shoulders, neck, stomach, and eventually your whole body. With practice, this stop-check-relax routine will take no more than a few seconds. Done regularly, it will reduce headaches and fatigue, and bring with it a more relaxed attitude.

### Deep relaxation

There are also lots of deep relaxation programmes, often involving tapes, which require at least half an hour a day of undisturbed solitude. There is an enormous range of books, tapes, and courses available, so when making a choice get a recommendation from someone whose opinion you trust.

### Meditation

Beyond relaxation is meditation. Many people are suspicious of meditation because of its religious overtones. However, research shows that it can be beneficial and does not have to be linked to any particular set of beliefs. A five-year study in the United States found that people who practice meditation suffer 50 percent less illness than non-meditators.

In essence, meditation involves concentrating your attention on one thing—a picture in the mind perhaps, a phrase, or sound. When other thoughts and images creep in, the meditator simply lets them go again.

### Breathing

Another element to relaxation is how you breathe. Rapid, shallow breathing can generate anxiety and eventually exhaustion. Exercises that teach us to breathe properly can therefore have a relaxing and invigorating effect. Once breathing is regular, our minds become free to wander, or to concentrate on positive images. Techniques that tap into this potential are often called guided imagery.

# looking
## AFTER YOURSELF

However holistic you make your home, unless you look after your own health, and that of those you live with, you will not receive the full benefit of the changes made to your living space.

Keeping well is about more than not getting sick. Achieving optimum health and fitness means choosing to live in a way that promotes these goals, rather than seeking a quick fix when you feel ill.

*Careful and proper preparation of wholesome food (RIGHT) is central to good health.*

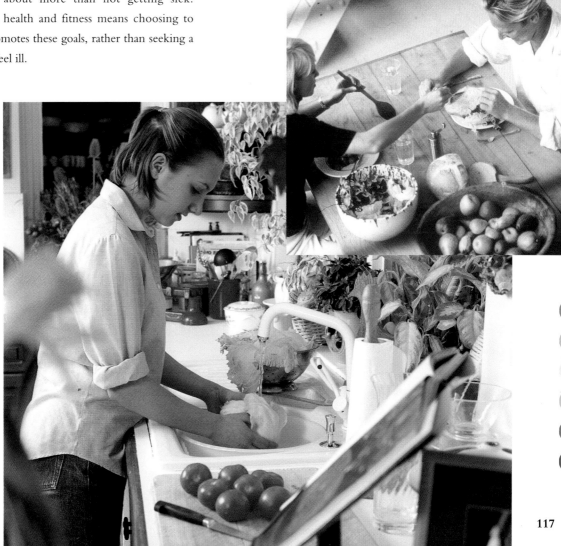

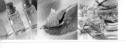

## FOOD HEALTH

Studies of the effect food has on health suggest that a sound diet is high in fiber and low in salt, sugar, and fat (particularly saturated fat), and is based on a wide variety of foods that will ensure delivery of all necessary nutrients.

An important part of good nutrition is food preparation. This in essence means buying organically grown and fresh produce, and then preparing it by steaming, stir frying, broiling, roasting, or stewing in preference to boiling, frying or deep-frying. Ideally, all food should be prepared and cooked just prior to consuming it.

Our throwaway culture has lost the art of storing food in a way that is hygienic, but which also makes it last longer in prime condition. However, if we are serious about what we eat and about reducing waste, it is time to possibly change some eating habits—shunning pre-packaged meals in favor of fresh produce—and to re-learn some of the old ways. Here are a few tips on food storage:

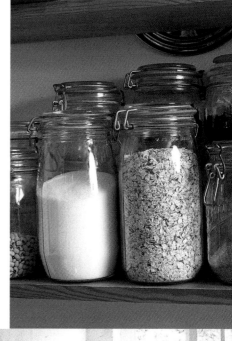

*To keep food safely, use glass containers with seals or lids (RIGHT), and store in cool place out of strong sunlight.*

+ Apples—arrange them in a single layer on trays.

+ Bread—store along with a slice of apple or potato to prevent the bread drying out too quickly.

+ Dairy products—these perish quickly and should be kept refrigerated. Eggs keep longest if stored thin end down, and cheese can be prevented from hardening if wrapped in a moist paper towel, then food wrap, and refrigerated.

+ Lemons—immerse them in a jar of cold water and leave in a refrigerator or cool larder.

+ Mushrooms—arrange them on a tray or plate, cover with damp paper towels and store in a refrigerator.

+ Potatoes—delay sprouting by storing them in a cool, dark place along with a couple of apples.

+ Soft fruit and salad vegetables—should be stored in a refrigerator. Cucumber and tomatoes, however, taste best if stored at room temperature. Maintain the crispness of scallions and celery by standing them in a tumbler of water, and watercress by immersing it in a bowl of water, and storing in a refrigerator.

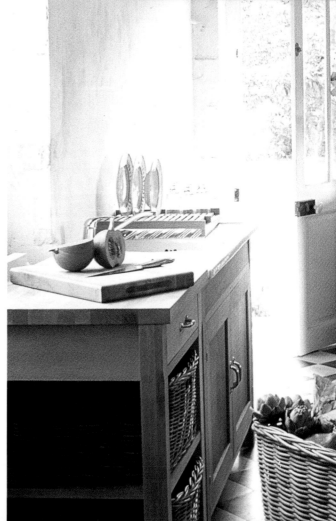

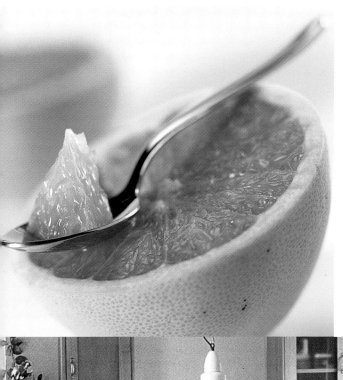

*Fresh organically produced foods (LEFT) should be part of our everyday diet.*

*A wonderful natural kitchen (BELOW) in which to store, prepare, and enjoy food.*

## TOXIC SUBSTANCES
*and food*

*A*ll trace elements are potentially toxic if ingested in high enough quantities, but toxic metals, such as lead, cadmium, mercury, aluminum, and copper, have well-documented deleterious effects on the body. To reduce the levels of these and other toxic substances: wash, clean, and wipe all food carefully being preparing it; avoid buying food that comes in unlined cans; avoid using aluminum pots and saucepans, foil, and food containing aluminum additives; and, if you are worried, have your water supply tested or use boiled or filtered water.

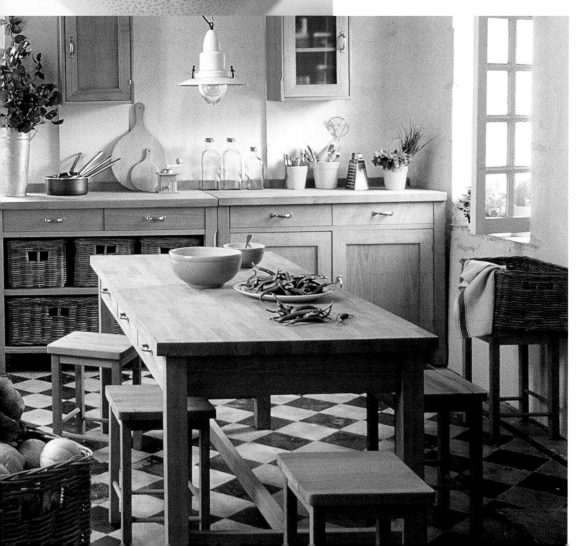

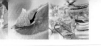

## ALLERGIES AND THE HOLISTIC HOME

The problem of allergies, and chemical and environmental sensitivities is a growing one, even though the causes of the allergies exist at very low levels. Indeed, over time, a sufferer may react adversely to smaller and smaller quantities of the "allergen."

If you are a chemically sensitive person it is important that your home is indeed your sanctuary. You should try to avoid any synthetic products in the home, or at least to reduce the load, as it were, by using natural products wherever possible. Any adaptations to your home should be attempted gradually—start by clearing out easier items such as chemically-based cleaning products, cosmetics, and clothes. Then tackle furnishings, structural problems, and household appliances. This process may take several years.

## EXERCISE AND LONG LIFE

Regular exercise will enhance and extend our active life, and help prevent and improve chronic conditions. Physiologically appropriate exercise can, for example, improve cardio-vascular function, skeletal muscle, tendons, and connective tissue, the skeleton itself, joints, metabolic functions, and psychological functioning.

Young and old alike need around 20 minutes of aerobic activity, three or four times a week. A realistic way of incorporating this naturally into your life is by taking a brisk 10 to 15 minute walk each day. Leave the car keys at home and walk to the shops, ignore the lift and take the stairs, or accompany someone on a dog-walking ramble through a park. Exercise done in this way is just as effective as hitting the gym.

## COMPLEMENTARY THERAPIES

Complementary medicine has been around in some form or other for centuries, often as the medicine of the people. It is tied in with folklore and tradition, and based on wisdom that has been passed down verbally from generation to generation. So there are many simple remedies that can be used in the home to treat common health problems. Complementary therapies, especially aromatherapy, Bach Flower Remedies, and crystals can also be used to invoke a positive and health-giving energy in your home.

There is a great variety of complementary therapies, but they do have some things in common. They all seek to mobilize the body's own self-healing capacities; they work at helping to rebalance the body rather than just suppress the symptoms; and therapists treat their clients as individuals and partners in the healing process, and deal with the client's problem in an integrated way, incorporating the social, psychological, emotional, and spiritual as well as the physical. Underlying these principles is a "world view," based on the belief in a life energy that is fundamental to a person's health and happiness.

> *The best recipe for health is to apply sweets scents to the brain.*

### Aromatherapy

Concentrated extracts from plants, called essential oils, are used by aromatherapists to tackle many common ailments. These essential oils, which are readily absorbed through the skin, appear to interact with your body pharmacologically, physiologically, and psychologically. One or two drops of these fragrant oils can also be added to a plant mister and sprayed around the home. Different rooms may require different oils. Lavender is a good oil for the living room to create a relaxing atmosphere, while geranium is a bedroom oil that fosters balance and harmony, for example.

Essential oils can be used in massage, skin oils and lotions, baths, douches, hot and cold compresses, flower waters, vaporization, and steam inhalation. As well as using essential oils, an aromatherapist will also look at exercise, diet, and other elements of a client's lifestyle that could be improved to enhance their health.

Essential oils can be safely used in the home provided instructions are followed carefully. They should never be taken internally, unless under the supervision of a qualified aromatherapist. There are also stringent guidelines for use during pregnancy or on children.

*A*romatherapy oils
have physical
and psychological
healing properties
beyond their health
and beauty uses.

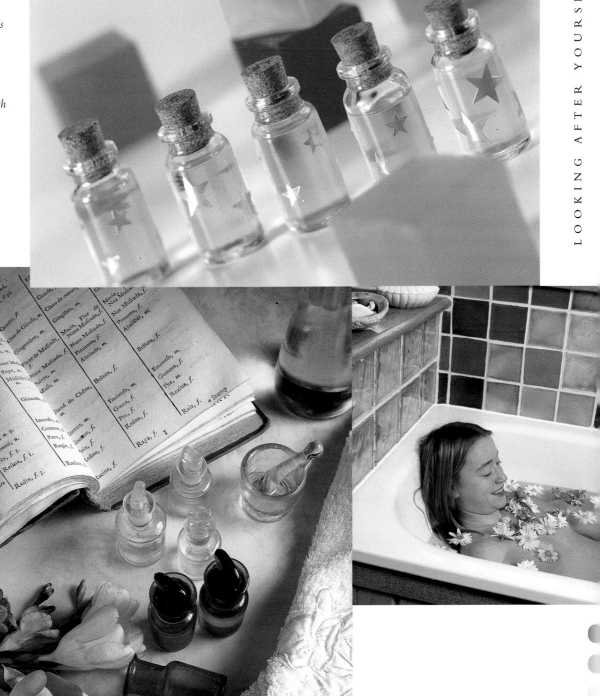

### Bach Flower Remedies

These remedies are made from 38 different species of wild flowers and were developed in the 1930s by a homeopathic physician, Dr Edward Bach. He argued that many diseases are caused by negative emotional states and personality problems. He selected flowers that he believed had special effects on the emotions and personality. A few drops of a remedy can be added to a plant mister filled with clear spring water and sprayed around the home to affect positively its subtle energies. Rescue Remedy will clear the after-effects of an argument, or cleanse a room where someone has been ill. To create a healthy, vital atmosphere, spray the home with Wild Rose.

### Homeopathy

The principle of homeopathy is that "like cures like." In effect, the same thing that causes a disease, if taken by a well person, will cure it in someone who is already sick. Samuel Hahnemann, the doctor who developed this therapy, found that the more dilute the remedy, the more effective it was. So only a few drops of a homeopathic tincture need to be added to water in a spray container to make an effective spray for the home. An arnica spray, for example, is used to counter the effects of a sudden shock or upset.

Homeopathic remedies come in a variety of forms, including tinctures, tablets, and powders. The remedy can be placed under the tongue, put into water and sipped, or put on a lactose tablet which is then dissolved in the mouth. With acute conditions there is normally a change after the first dose, but chronic conditions will take longer to treat. A remedy should not continue to be taken once an improvement has been noted. Remedies should be taken at least 10 to 15 minutes after eating, and no food or strong-tasting drink ingested immediately after taking a remedy. It is always best to seek advice from a qualified homeopath before taking any remedy.

### Herbal medicine

This ancient form of medicine uses plants to promote healing and maintain health. Many drugs were developed from plants, but whereas conventional medicine seeks to isolate the "active ingredient," herbal medicine uses remedies made from the whole plant.

Herbalists argue that the natural chemical balance of a whole plant has a more holistic effect. Any herbal remedy prescribed by a herbalists will usually be accompanied by a discussion of diet, exercise, and lifestyle. Chemists and health food shops also sell herbal remedies, and loose herbs are available from herbal suppliers.

### Massage

A good massage does more that simply unknot muscles—it can relax and "heal" the body to such an extent that "passageways" of free thought can be opened. It is as though the act of untying and de-stressing the body makes it easier to think clearly, therefore making it possible to sort important issues from irrelevancies.

Something that older people in particular, often comment upon is the lack of physical affection they receive. One practical way to address this is to give or receive a massage. It does not have to be a full body massage—a simple hand massage can be extraordinarily effective in relieving tension and, equally importantly, reconnecting us to the rest of the human race.

*Complementary therapies, like massage, will mobilize the body's capacity for self-healing.*

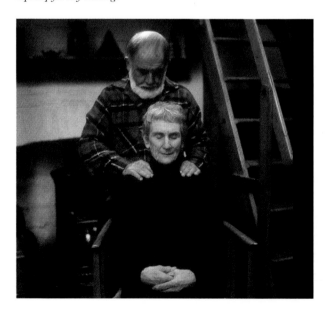

## Neck and shoulder massage

This massage will relieve a tension headache, and can be done through clothes. The person receiving the massage should sit in a chair with a low back that leaves the upper back and neck free.

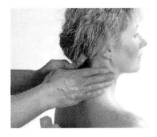

**1** Sit the recipient in the chair and stand behind it. Place your hands on each side of the neck.

**2** Making contact mostly with the palm of the hand, start at the top and stroke, with moderate pressure, down the neck. Continue the movement to the shoulders.

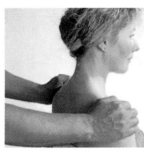

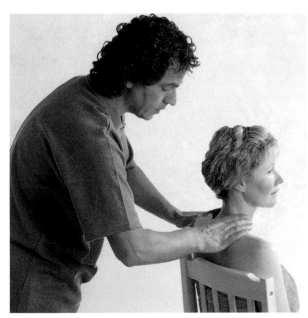

**3** As you go over the top of the shoulders, use the fingers as well as the palms to increase the pressure slightly. When your hands reach the outside of the shoulders, return to the top of the neck without losing contact with the skin. Repeat several times maintaining a slow rhythm.

**4** Place one hand on each shoulder as shown. Gently apply pressure with the thumb of each as you move it toward the top of the shoulder.

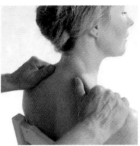
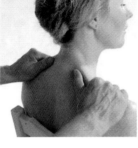

**6** Stand to one side of the recipient. Place one hand midway along the top of the furthest shoulder. Gently lift and squeeze the muscle between the fingertips and the heel of the hand.

**5** Apply a gentle squeeze with the fingers and palm. Raise the thumb as it nears the fingers to avoid pinching the skin. Repeat several times, increasing the pressure.

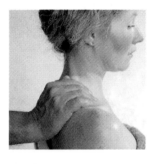

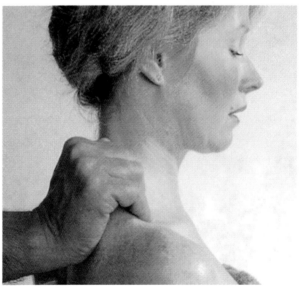

**7** Continue to squeeze, letting the heel of the hand move toward the fingertips so as to stretch the muscle across its fibers. Repeat several times, then repeat for the other shoulder.

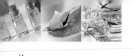

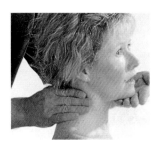

**8** Stand at the side of the recipient and support the chin. Place the other at the back of the neck as shown. Compress the neck muscles gently between fingers and thumb.

**9** Continue with the compression as you begin to stretch the muscles and overlying skin away from the spine. Ease the pressure as the hands begins to slide away.

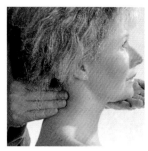

**10** Place one hand at the back of the neck with the thumb just behind one ear, the middle finger in the same position under the other ear.

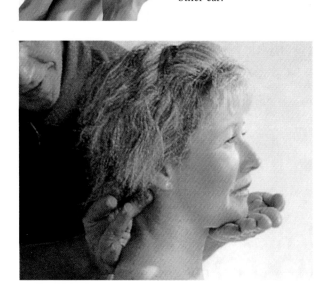

**11** Apply light pressure equally with the thumb and middle fingers as you run them toward the midpoint of the neck. As the thumb and finger meet, lift off, and return to original positions. Repeat several times.

## Aromatherapy hand massage

You can do this massage without oil, or make a massage oil by mixing together one tablespoon of almond oil and two teaspoons of an essential oil. People have strong preferences when it comes to smell, so let the receiver choose which oil you use. To start, ask the recipient of the massage to sit comfortably. Throughout the massage, make sure that one of your hands is supporting the hand being massaged.

**1** Hold the recipient's hand palm up and stroke the palm with the heel of your hand. Push down toward their wrist and then slowly glide back to your starting point.

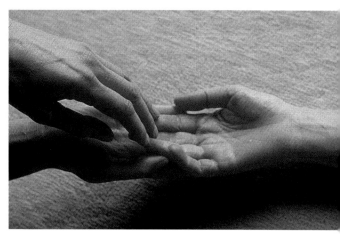

**2** Turn the hand over and support it with the fingers of both your hands. Stroke the back of the hand with your thumbs, from the knuckles to wrist. Stroke slowly toward the wrist with your fingers and thumb. Pull back firmly to stretch the hand.

**3** Hold the hand palm down. Stroke each finger from the tip to knuckle, then squeeze it all over. Apply a gentle pressure with your thumb around each joint, and then stretch each finger gently to ease the joints. Massage the thumb deeply.

**4** To finish, stroke the whole hand and then sandwich it between yours and hold quietly for a few seconds. Release the pressure and slide your hands slowly off, repeat this a couple of times. Repeat the whole sequence with the recipient's other hand.

# HOLISTIC *first aid box*

*The following not only gives you an idea of what an holistic first aid box could contain, but it also shows that there are natural remedies for many ailments of the body and the spirit. These products should be stored as carefully as any medicine.*

✦ ALOE VERA GEL—TO SOOTHE MINOR BURNS OR SUNBURN.

✦ ARNICA CREAM—APPLY TO BRUISES AND SPRAINS.

✦ CALENDULA (MARIGOLD) CREAM—AN ANTISEPTIC AND ANTIFUNGAL CREAM FOR CUTS, GRAZES, AND DRY SKIN.

✦ CAMOMILE TEA—FOR INSOMNIA.

✦ CHICKWEED CREAM—FOR DRAWING SPLINTERS, BOILS, AND INSECT STINGS.

✦ ECHINACEA CAPSULES—FOR COLDS AND 'FLU.

✦ HOMEOPATHIC ARNICA 6C TABLETS—TO COUNTER THE EFFECTS OF SHOCK.

✦ HOMEOPATHIC APIS 6C—FOR INSECT STINGS.

✦ LAVENDER ESSENTIAL OIL—RUB ON TEMPLES FOR HEADACHES, APPLY TO BURNS AND SCALDS, AND ADD TO BATHS FOR A RELAXING SOAK.

✦ NUX VOMICA 6C—FOR IRRITABLE HEADACHES FROM OVER-INDULGENCE IN CAFFEINE, ALCOHOL, OR RICH FOOD, AND WHEN STUDYING INTENSIVELY.

✦ PEPPERMINT TEA—FOR INDIGESTION.

✦ BACH'S RESCUE REMEDY—TO COUNTER SHOCK, AND NERVOUS UPSETS.

✦ SLIPPERY ELM TABLETS—FOR INDIGESTION AND STOMACH UPSETS.

✦ TEA-TREE ESSENTIAL OIL—AN ANTISEPTIC AND ANTIFUNGAL OIL FOR CUTS AND GRAZES, AND WHEN ADDED TO A BATH WILL HELP TREAT COLDS AND 'FLU.

*Watching a herbal tea seep is a lesson in patience. Enjoying its fragrance and palate, the reward.*

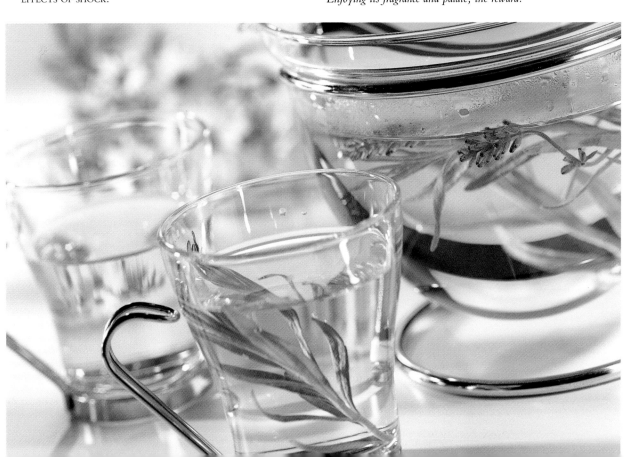

# INDEX

# A C K N O W L E D G M E N T S

The Publishers would like to thank the following for opening their homes and for all their valuable help—Tony and Christian Lewin, Sally Cox at the Michael Hall School, Christina Korth and her beautiful kindergarten at Michael Hall, and to Rebecca Dewing for impromptu modeling. Thanks also to Barbara Douglas, Susan Marfleet, Fiona Taylor, and to Leslie Kyle for sourcing photographs in Australia.

Thanks also to the following for lending furnishings and decorations for photography—Anna French for fabrics (page 83, *bl*); Derek Small at Colours Clothing and Craft, Farnham, Surrey (UK 01252 733 476) Purves & Purves, London  (UK 0171 580 8223)—tower lamp (page 42, *tl*), wool rug (page 94, *d*), wooden mouse (page 95, *cr*), Alison white mulberry screen ( page 104, *t*); The Pier,  London (UK 0171 814 5020).

## PICTURE CREDITS

(*l*-left; *r*-right; *t*-top; *c*-centre; *b*-bottom)
P2—Malabar (*tl*); p4—Habitat (*tl*), Ikea (*cr*), Malabar (*bl*); p5—Ikea (*c*); p7—Iron Design Company★ (*tr*), Malabar (*bl*)

### Section 1
P11—Peter Bateman Photography, Aust (*l*); p12—Interior Archive (*l*), Habitat (*tc*, *br*), Peter Bateman Photography, Aust (*tr*), Fired Earth (*bc*); p13—Habitat (*c*, *b*);  p17—Wools of New Zealand (*t*), Kährs (*b*); p18—Peter Bateman Photography, Aust; p19—Pergo Laminate Flooring★★ (*b*);  p27—Malabar (*t*);  p28—Patti McConville, Image Bank (*l*);  p31—Malabar (*tl*);  p32—Wools of New Zealand (*br*);  p34—Iron Design Company★ (*b*);  p37—Ikea;  p39—Habitat (*tr*);  p41—Peter Bateman Photography, Aust (*t*);  p44—Pergo Laminate Flooring ★★ (*l*), Iron Design Company★ (*r*);  p45—Kährs (*br*);  p 47—Wools of New Zealand (*tl*);  p53—Malabar;  p56—Malabar (*t*), Peter Bateman Photography, Aust (*b*)

### Section 2
P62—Kährs;  p63—Pergo Laminate Flooring ★★ (*t*, *b*); p64—Kährs (*t*), Pergo Laminate Flooring★★ (*b*); p65—Malabar (*t*); p66/67—Multiyork Furniture Limited; p68—Peter Bateman Photography, Aust (*tr*); p71—Malabar (*t*); p72—Habitat (*d*, *b*, *tr*), Casa Paints (*cr*); p73—Habitat (*c*), Fired Earth (*b*); p75—Habitat (*t*); p76—Ikea (*b*); p77—Ikea; p81—Ikea; p82—Designed Blinds, Aust (*t*); p84—Ikea; p85—Wools of New Zealand; p86—Kährs (*b*); p87—Futon Company; p88—Futon Company (*b*); p89—Pergo Laminate Flooring★★ (*bl*), The Pier (*cr*); p90—Futon Company; p94—Habitat (*t*); p95—Habitat (*tr*); p96—Wools of New Zealand (*t*); p98—Armitage Shanks Limited (*b*); p99—Ikea (*d*); p105—Ikea (*b*); p108—Peter Bateman Photography, Aust (*b*); p109—Peter Bateman Photography, Aust (*cr*); p111—Habitat (*tl*).

### Section3
P114 Iron Design Company★; p117—Wools of New Zealand (*t*); p118—Habitat (*b*); p122 and 124 (*r*)—Fausto Dorelli from the *Book of Massage* (1984), by permission of Gaia Books Ltd. London.

★Copyright & Design belong to the Iron Design Company and no reproduction of the photographs or the designs is permitted without permission of The Iron Design Company.

★★ Pergo Laminate Flooring – contact 0800 374771 or www.pergo.com for stockists.

Abode Interiors Photography and Library— p2 *tr* Andreas von Einsiedel, *br* Ian Parry; p7 *tl* Ian Parry, *br* Ian Parry; p10 Ian Parry; p12 *d* Ian Parry; p13 *t* Ian Parry; p15 Ian Parry; p20 Ian Parry; p21 *bl* Ian Parry; p22 Ian Parry; p23 *t* Brian Harrison; p24 *t* Ian Parry, *c* Ian Parry; p25 Ian Parry ; p33 *t* Ian Parry; p36 Ian Parry; p40 *t* Trevor Richards; p42 *b* David Parmiter; p43 *b* Ian Parry; p50 *b* Ian Parry; p57 *t* Ian Parry; p59 *l* Trevor Richards; p60 *t* Chris Grayson, *b* Ian Parry; p68 *tl* Ian Parry, *cr* Ian Parry, *bl* Ian Parry , *br* Ian Parry; p69 Ian Parry; p72 *tl* Ian Parry; p73 *t* Ian Parry; p74 Ian Parry; p75 *tr* Ian Parry, *b* Ian Parry; p76 *tr* Ian Parry; p78 *t* Ian Parry, *b* Ian Parry; p79 *tr* Trevor Richards, *b* Chris Grayson; p80 Andreas von Einsiedel; p86 *t* Ian Parry; p88 *t* Trevor Richards, *c* Trevor Richards; p89 *tr* Andreas von Einsiedel; p93 *tl* Ian Parry, *b* Ian Parry; p97 Andreas von Einsiedel; p99 *tr* Trevor Richards, *cr* Ian Parry, *bl* David Parmiter; p100 *b* Ian Parry; p101 *t* Ian Parry; p106 Ian Parry; p107 *l* Ian Parry, *br* Ian Parry; p108 *t* Ian Parry; p109 *br* Ian Parry.

Elizabeth Whiting & Associates—p2 *bl*; p3 Rodney Hyett; p4 *tr* Di Lewis; p8 *tr* Di Lewis; p10 *l* Neil Lorimer; p12 *cr* Neil Lorimer; p19 *t* Michael Dunne; p24 *b* Di Lewis; p41 Tommy Candler; p49 Tommy Candler; p51 *t* Spike Powell; p52 *b*; p57 Karl-Dietrich Buhler; p59 *t* Friedhelm Thomas, *br* Peter Wolosynski; p65 *b* Simon Upton; p70 Jerry Tubby; p76 *l* Julian Nieman; p82 Di Lewis; p83 *d* Michael Dunne; p96 *b* Dennis Stone; p98 *c* Rodney Hyett; p99 *tl* Tim Street-Porter, *bl* Tom Leighton; *tr* Di Lewis; p101 *b* Debi Treloar; p103 Jerry Harpur; p105 *tr* Rodney Hyett; p107 *tr*; p109 *tr* Karl-Dietrich Buhler, *d/bl* Jerry Harpur; p110 Di Lewis; p113 Mari O'Hara; p115 b Jerry Tubby; p116 Jerry Harpur.